An Introduction to Medical Leadership for Surgeons

Stanley Zackary Trooskin

An Introduction to Medical Leadership for Surgeons

Maximizing Interpersonal Interactions for Success

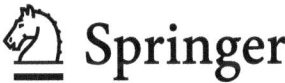 Springer

Stanley Zackary Trooskin
Department of Surgery Rutgers Robert Wood
Johnson Medical School
New Brunswick, NJ, USA

ISBN 978-3-031-44263-6   ISBN 978-3-031-44264-3   (eBook)
https://doi.org/10.1007/978-3-031-44264-3

This Springer imprint is published by the registered company Springer Nature Switzerland AG
The registered company address is: Gewerbestrasse 11, 6330 Cham, Switzerland

Paper in this product is recyclable.

Acknowledgements

The author would like to thank those friends who supplied advice and support. I have been blessed to work with fabulous administrative assistants that helped me get through every day's challenges of balancing my busy practice and administrative responsibilities. In Philadelphia, I was helped by the multitalented Ms. Mary Baxter. In New Brunswick, I was supported by the late Ms. Selma Zimmeran, Ms. Carol Squindo, and Ms. Leala May, whose loyalty over the last 2 decades was greatly appreciated. Special thanks to my colleague, Dr. Andrew Roberts, who has given me 30 years of support and most lately enthusiastic encouragement on the potential value of this work. Mr. Vince Joseph, who teaches leadership skills, helped me improve each chapter with specific suggestions. Dr. Jacob Moalem reviewed an early draft and offered insightful comments on the central theme.

I would like to dedicate this book to my family. My three forgiving daughters, Stacey, Gerri, and Amy, now incredibly successful, who when growing up tolerated to a greater or lesser degree my jammed packed professional life. Most recently they encouraged me throughout this recent writing process. Most of all, I would like to thank my longstanding life partner, Estelle, who has been at my side since 1970. She was there for every adventure and whose frequently needed advice kept me grounded and on track. Without her unending support, cheerleading, and dedication to our family, I would not have had much success at all.

Contents

About the Author

Stanley Zackary Trooskin, MD had a 42-year career as a busy clinical general surgeon. After obtaining an undergraduate degree from Rutgers University, he attended the University of Pittsburgh School of Medicine. He trained in general surgery at New York University Bellevue Medical Center. He spent his career in New Brunswick, New Jersey at Rutgers Robert Wood Johnson Medical School (formerly University of Medicine and Dentistry Robert Wood Johnson Medical School), in Brooklyn at SUNY Downstate and the Kings County Hospital Center, and in Philadelphia at Drexel University College of Medicine (formerly Medical College of Pennsylvania) and the Medical College of Pennsylvania and Hahnemann Hospitals. Dr. Trooskin had multiple successful leadership experiences as trauma director and in service chief and chair positions. He also had roles as medical staff president and as chief medical officer. Dr. Trooskin recently retired from surgical practice and now resides with his wife and extended family in Philadelphia, where he writes about his experiences and coaches baseball skills in a Rookie League for 8-year-olds.

Chapter 1
Introduction

In our present complex health care climate, there is a need for clinicians who understand excellence in patient care to participate in leadership positions. Some successful clinicians have a good understanding of what patients and their providers need
to obtain the best possible outcomes. These providers need to be more involved with
their administrative partners to deliver clinical care with excellent access and outcomes. How do we train these clinicians to also be successful in medical administration? As I looked back on my long clinical and administrative career, I was struck
with the thought that, for me, quality surgical training was the starting point for my
medical leadership training. As a well-trained, successful clinical surgeon, I had to
be very good at self-questioning and striving for continuous improvement. My
experience has taught me that this same skill set was also essential in my becoming
a medical leader. My leadership training was based on this type of trial-and-error
learning, analyzing what I was doing that was working or not working as I was trying to lead my team. Is there a better way to develop medical leaders?

Medical leadership courses are now widely available. I participated in my first
medical leadership course at the age of 65 years. The course was created by our
university hospital's recently retired Chief Operating Officer. As he started the next
phase of his career teaching medical administration at Rutgers University, one of his
first assignments was to develop a medical leadership course for the up-and-coming
next generation of Robert Wood Johnson University Hospital's medical staff leaders. At the time, I was the longstanding Chief of the hospital's Surgical Services. I
interpreted my invitation as more of a courtesy. I did not fit the typical "student
profile." I was not a member of the next generation of hospital leaders. I suspect I
was chosen because in my role as one of the senior medical staff leaders, my presence would add balance and credibility to the class.

I found the course to be utterly fascinating. The topics covered all the standard
elements that every excellent medical leadership course should include. There were
historical references to great leaders in other disciplines, such as Abraham Lincoln.
We analyzed all the chapters in the book, *Good to Great*, by Collins [1]. The course

S. Z. Trooskin, *An Introduction to Medical Leadership for Surgeons*,
https://doi.org/10.1007/978-3-031-44264-3_1

presented, in depth, the topic of emotional intelligence as an essential characteristic of effective leadership [2]. We learned about Myers-Briggs testing for personality traits and styles [3]. The basics of hospital finances and business accounting systems were also studied. We met once a week for 7 weeks, and I enjoyed every minute, including the homework assignments.

I was very impressed that this formal training in medical leadership had validated the operational techniques I had learned and practiced daily throughout my long career. I realized the lessons that I learned very gradually, via trial-and-error experiences, helped me to succeed during my surgical residency, especially as a chief resident. My personal experiences also helped me in building and administering a successful referral practice, starting and directing trauma centers, serving as chief of surgery at university hospitals, and functioning as an interim department chair, medical staff president, and chief medical officer for large academic medical centers. In short, without having taken any leadership courses, I had learned and employed the basic principles now routinely taught in medical leadership courses. It was learning the hard way.

As I started to think about my slow yet steady development as a medical leader, my first conclusion was that I was incredibly grateful for my surgical training, which instilled in me the importance of lifelong learning. Surgical training taught me to always try to analyze my outcomes to discover ways to improve them. This started with the attendance at the Surgical Morbidity and Mortality Conference (M&M). I believe that honest self-reflection can be readily demonstrated in the weekly effective M&M conferences and was an early crucial step for my professional development. It was where I had first learned to effectively analyze events that had gone poorly and to decide what I was going to do better next time. If you can learn these lessons well as a surgeon and then apply this concept combined with self-awareness and empathy to personal interactions in the hospital, clinics, and administrative suites, you can also have remarkable success as a medical leader. I, therefore, believe that excellent surgical training combined with emotional intelligence can be the starting point for a career in medical leadership.

The educational process of trial and error, identifying what worked and did not work, and my ability to self-correct had served me well. Nonetheless, it is also obvious to me that there are great benefits to be accrued by participating in medical leadership courses. It should be more efficient than trial-and-error learning to prepare surgeons for leadership as they progress through their careers. It is better not to leave medical leadership education to trial and error. It is too slow and inefficient.

My review of the literature [4–7] revealed that one leadership course may be able to change and improve an individual's leadership capabilities. That raises an issue to consider: Is one medical leadership course enough? General Mark Hertling pointed out that training in certain disciplines, such as for the military [8], occurs at multiple levels during the maturation of the developing leader. Training in medical leadership should not necessarily end after one course. Medical leadership courses can be helpful in developing the skills needed for success at all levels of career development. One solitary course targeting mid-level medical providers is not a realistic approach to creating effective long-term medical leaders for the future. At various levels of one's career, the issues faced are different, and the leadership courses should be tailored to deal with those issues. In fact, medical leadership should probably begin in medical school and residency training and be continued throughout one's surgical career. The focus of the courses should be directed to the surgeon's career level. I know I would have made fewer errors and had more initial successes if I had had a better idea of what would work before I made the avoidable errors.

The principles of good medical leadership have been well-defined. The application of those principles at the different levels of training has not. As I look back on my career, I have come to conclude that there may be benefits in describing how those leadership principles can be applied at different levels of experience. There is a common thread applicable to medical leaders at all levels of a surgeon's career. That thread is the application of emotional intelligence to all aspects of medical leadership. Specific issues regarding leadership and the application of emotional intelligence will be different for the surgical resident, the newly minted surgical attending who must deal with establishing a practice, interacting with colleagues, and dealing with senior associates. Likewise, learning to lead while developing a new program will require another set of applications of emotional intelligence and leadership skills. The same is true for interacting with colleagues outside the surgical disciplines and getting multidisciplinary teams to function smoothly. As the years go by, successful surgeons may find themselves as formal or informal leaders in their hospitals. For each of these levels, the principles remain the same, but the specific applications to getting the "team" to achieve those common goals may be very different.

I investigated the literature to see if it would be possible to give a complete evidence-based discussion and compile advice on medical leadership for surgeons at various career stages. Unfortunately, there is a dearth of scientific evidence and advice specifically for surgeons as their careers progress. The purpose of this current effort is to attempt to introduce leadership training to the various stations in a surgeon's career by focusing on the concept of emotional intelligence and the surgeon's interpersonal interactions. I have therefore included suggestions for success that I learned the "hard way" that may be helpful to the surgical resident for practice building, operating team function, and at various other leadership positions.

This short book is not intended to be a complete guide to medical leadership for surgeons but an introduction to some basic concepts and recommendations that may prove to be helpful to surgeons at various stages of their careers. I offer no specific detailed advice on dealing with the financial issues that abound in medicine today but focus on the personal interactions and relationships that are essential for success in medical leadership for surgeons. This book is a compilation of anecdotal stories and lessons learned from my experiences as a medical leader that links those lessons to the current basic principles of medical leadership and the application of emotional intelligence. I volunteer that I do not have all the medical leadership answers that surgeons will need over the course of their careers. I've had my share of successes and failures, some of which were calamitous. I will not spare the reader my experiences that did not work so that it will also be possible to learn what not to do.

The structure will be an introduction to the basic principles of medical leadership followed by their application at various career stages. I will focus on the specific lessons for medical leadership relevant to surgical residents, junior attending surgeons establishing a practice, for those developing and building new programs, for new division chiefs or chairs, and for those undertaking hospital leadership positions, such as medical staff officers and hospital administration.

References

1. Collins J. Good to great. New York: Random House; 2001.
2. Goleman D. Emotional intelligence. 25th ed. New York: Bantam Books; 2020.
3. Myers I. The Myers Briggs type indicator: manual. Sunnyvale: Consulting Psychologists Press; 1962.
4. Straus SE, Soobiah C, Levinson W. The impact of leadership training programs on physicians in academic medical centers: a systematic review. Acad Med. 2013;88(5):710–23.
5. Lyons O, Su'a B, Locke M, Hill A. A systematic review of leadership training for medical students. N Z Med J. 2018;131(1468):75–84.
6. Simpson C, Silberberg M, Hibbard ST, Lyn MJ, Sawin G. Perceived benefits of training clinicians in community engagement for a leadership development program. Fam Med. 2022;54(2):134–8.
7. Center for Creative Leadership (www.ccl.org).
8. Hertling M. Growing physician leaders. New York: Rosetta Books; 2016.

Chapter 2
Basic Principles of Medical Leadership

The basic principles of leadership, taught in every good medical leadership course, are straightforward. The most important concept is to use emotional intelligence when dealing with everyone. This holds whether leading a few individuals or leading large groups. It also applies to leading in all directions. Leading those who report to you is termed "leading down." Leading those who are designated as your peers, whose help you need to be successful, is termed "leading sideways." Getting the people who the leader reports to involved and on board with the plan is known as "leading up."

A good leader will consistently demonstrate emotional intelligence. One can never know who is watching and listening to the leader's behavior. Emotional intelligence involves dealing with people with honesty, respect, and caring behavior. It is the application of self-awareness, self-discipline, and empathy. Emotional Intelligence is the ability to make your emotions work for you by using them in ways that produce the results you have been seeking. Daniel Goleman and Associates [1] concluded that emotional intelligence was the number one predictor of a leader's success. It is not a skill that should be exhibited episodically. General Mark Hertling, in his book *Growing Physician Leaders*, underscores the importance of demonstrating character. Continuously demonstrating good character (via emotional intelligence) is the critical ingredient for great success as a medical leader.

Bruce Flareau and J. M. Bohn [2] refer to the six Ps of Physician Leadership. They contend that mastering these principles will lead to the development of excellent leaders in medicine. The six Ps are People, Presence, Politics, Process, Perspective, and Principles of Business. I recommend this monograph as a primer of the basic principles. To a large degree, the concepts that they elucidate under the People and Presence are about dealing with people with emotional intelligence: being thoughtful, kind, and listening attentively while understanding and considering others' opinions and encouraging input.

Stewart Gabel [3] has summarized the linkage between power and leadership as well as discussed Raven's [4, 5] concepts of power and the physician's potential for

S. Z. Trooskin, *An Introduction to Medical Leadership for Surgeons*, https://doi.org/10.1007/978-3-031-44264-3_2

influence: "Power and leadership are linked via the personal characteristics and competencies of the leader." The different concepts of power that are available for physicians to consider while practicing surgery and in the arena of medical leadership are well delineated in this paper. Raven defined leadership as involving "working in socially appropriate ways to influence others in subordinate or follower positions to achieve principle-driven goals and objectives that these individuals may not have wanted to reach, may not have thought of reaching, or may not have had the courage or motivation to attempt on their own." Raven also defined the six primary bases of power: (1) Legitimate or positional power, (2) Expert power, (3) Informational power, (4) Reward power, (5) Coercive power, and (6) Referent power. One can see that physicians as leaders can exert their influence and power in ways that utilize many of these. Chief residents will have positional, reward, and potentially coercive power over their resident team members. Division Chiefs and Chairs will have all of those plus expert and perhaps referential power.

Others [6] have outlined a system of classifying different leadership styles and incorporating the concept of power. A transactional style employs rewards and punishments. A charismatic leader relies on a style of communicating in a moving, enthusiastic, and emotional way. These types of leaders can express their vision to inspire others to trust and follow them. They can express their views with social sensitivity and connect with their teams. A situational leadership style is one that directs the team members and sells or convinces them of the plan and delegates freely. This type of style employs delegation with limited leader input. It can also refer to applying a style of leadership that fits a given situation. For example, a code team may function best with a transactional leader during the actual code.

The final leadership style is called transformational. The transformational leader shares the leadership process with the team members and employs intellectual stimulation, treats the individual with consideration, employs inspirational motivation, and acts as a role model. Bernard Bass and his collaborators [7, 8] described the characteristics and activities of the transformational leader. This includes idealized influence or one that is based on principles or an organization's mission-driven vision for the future. By employing inspirational motivation, the leader displays the qualities of "conviction, dedication, energy and optimism." Using intellectual stimulation, the leader empowers and challenges his team members to find or create better solutions. The transformational leader treats his team members as individuals and has an interest in their growth and development. They occupy the role of mentor. Simply put, this type of leader consistently demonstrates excellent emotional intelligence and great character.

Sari Huikko-Tarvainen [9] performed a qualitative study in Finland of a group of 50 physicians at various levels including residents, fellows, chiefs, and department chairs to delineate the elements of good physician leadership. These physicians valued "trust, fairness, empathy, social skills, two-way communication skills, regular feedback, collegial respect and emotional intelligence." In short, they wanted their leaders to have medical expertise and good manners. They should, in all aspects of their behavior, demonstrate character or emotional intelligence.

One of the aspects of being successful as a leader is to get things done, to make progress. Quoting one of my leadership mentors, Mr. Vince Joseph: "Are you an owner or a renter?" Meaning: Is this project important to you, or are you just putting in the time? Successful surgeons understand that question. In clinical care, the surgeon is responsible for the ultimate results. Historically, we referred to the surgeon as the "Captain of the Ship." There is no truly successful surgeon who hides from their outcomes. If you want a surgical career noted for outstanding clinical results, the total assumption of the ultimate responsibility is the most important requirement.

That translates well to project management and monitoring progress. There should be self-employment of open-eyed evaluation for progress. The surgeon as a leader needs to assess the barriers to success and have a plan to overcome them. Career advancement in medical leadership is based on a track record of success. Only "owners" have long-term successful careers in medical leadership.

Jim Collins, in his book *Good to Great*, presents the characteristics and principles followed by companies/businesses with a history of multiple generational, long-term, sustained success. He describes his research on companies that have gone from being good to consistently great. The great companies have what he describes as Level 5 leaders, who are a "paradoxical blend of personal humility and professional will." He refers to getting the right people on the bus and the wrong ones off the bus and getting the correct team members in the right seats on that bus. It takes a culture of discipline to be successful. The Collins book is timeless and should be studied carefully by nascent leaders.

The surgical leader should understand that it is their responsibility to build and maintain the culture of discipline. Goleman and associates underscore that the most crucial aspect of emotional intelligence is self-awareness. Those who have great self-awareness can read and understand their own emotions. They are realistic about their own strengths and weaknesses and can accept criticism. They know when they do not know all the answers and when to ask for help. They will welcome contrary opinions, realizing that is the best way to stay out of trouble. Those with high emotional intelligence can exhibit self-confidence without demonstrating arrogance.

References

1. Goleman D, Boyatzis R, McKee A. Primal leadership. Boston: Harvard Business Review Press; 2013.
2. Flareau B, Bohn J. The six P's of physician leadership: a primer for emerging and developing leaders. Ft. Myers: Kumu Press; 2013.
3. Gabel S. Power, leadership and transformation: the doctor's potential for influence. Med Educ. 2012;46(12):1152–60.
4. Raven BH. Social power and compliance in health care. In: Maes S, Spielberger S, Defares CD, Sararson IG, editors. Topics in health psychology. New York: John Wiley & Sons; 1988. p. 229–44.
5. Raven BH. The bases of power and the power/interaction model of interpersonal influence. Anal Soc Issues Public Policy. 2008;8(1):1–22.
6. AdventHealth Online (www.adventhealth.com), July 27, 2020.

7. Bass BM. The handbook of leadership: theory, research and managerial applications. 4th ed. New York: Free Press; 2008.
8. Bass BM. Two decades of research and development in transformational leadership. Eur J Work Organ Psychol. 1999;1:9–32.
9. Huikko-Tarvainen S. Elements of perceived good physician leadership and their relation to leadership theory. Leadersh Health Serv (Bradf Engl). 2021:14–29. ahead-of-print(ahead-of-print)

Chapter 3
Leadership for Surgical Residents: Effective Clinical Team Leading

Most people consider leaders in medicine to be department chairs, division chiefs, or physicians functioning in hospital or medical school administrative roles. In fact, surgeons begin as leaders during the residency training years. They start leading teams on rounds by participating in resuscitation, code, and trauma teams. Chief residents will be leading their services daily. Later, they will lead teams in the operating room and will lead their practices in the many aspects of patient care. There is no better time to start leadership training than residency so that lessons learned there can applied throughout their careers.

What should surgical residents know about leadership? First, they should be introduced to the importance of demonstrating character and that their character is always on display. They should begin to apply the principles and domains of emotional intelligence. They should also learn the importance of not only leading their teams but also leading their peers by functioning effectively in multidisciplinary teams. This will be illustrated by some of my personal experiences.

I had my first opportunity to closely observe a surgical leader as a newly minted intern, or as the position is now known, a post-medical school graduate year 1 (PGY-1). My first leaders were my chief residents. The team members, including me, were constantly observing him on rounds and in the operating room. I had been assigned to Bellevue Hospital Medical Center, a large inner-city hospital, for my very first rotation. I noted initially that my chief resident dealt with his patients with compassion. He also always generally behaved like a gentleman. I could see the emotion on his face when he was pleased with an outcome, or when he was not pleased. When things did not go well, I could easily appreciate the apprehension and concern in his eyes and voice. I also noticed that at times there was some inconsistency in his behavior.

One occasion was particularly illustrative. A patient presented with a small bowel obstruction, and my chief elected to attempt nonoperative management. That lasted a few days, until our X-ray conference with the attending surgeons. The patient had not improved after several days and continued to have the classic

S. Z. Trooskin, *An Introduction to Medical Leadership for Surgeons*, https://doi.org/10.1007/978-3-031-44264-3_3

radiographic findings of complete small bowel obstruction. With the attending surgeon's influence, immediately following the conclusion of the conference, the patient was taken to the operating room, where he was found to have a gangrenous (frankly black and dead) small bowel. He required a small bowel resection. He subsequently did not do well.

The Morbidity and Mortality Conference for this case, one of my first, was eye opening for me. The chief resident presented the details of the case factually. When asked what he would do differently the next time a similar situation arose, he attributed the poor outcome to the fact that the patient was not given preoperative antibiotics. The responsibility for ordering the antibiotics belonged to one of the other interns. As I sat in the conference, I was concerned that my chief resident did not mention the major clinical error: There was a delay in operating on this patient who clinically presented with complete small bowel obstruction. Although the lack of antibiotics may possibly have contributed to the outcome, the most important major contributing factor to the poor outcome was the delay in performing the operation. I was disappointed that my chief did not publicly take full responsibility for the actions of his team and for his decision to delay the operation.

A few months later, while rotating at the Manhattan Veterans Hospital, I was exposed to a different style of leadership by another chief resident. He was quite confident in his abilities and very dogmatic. He ran his service with a very strict, demanding, almost militaristic style with employment of the chain of command. He expected us to pay attention to every detail, which in terms of clinical care is an excellent strategy. However, if a detail was missed, one would learn about it in front of the entire team on morning or afternoon rounds. All deviance from what he expected was met with public sharp criticism.

I remember one patient who presented with colon cancer. He had a long history of smoking two packs of cigarettes a day for over 30 years and clearly had chronic obstructive pulmonary disease (COPD). His preoperative arterial blood gas revealed a well-compensated, chronic respiratory acidosis. His arterial pO_2 was 62 mmHg, which was very low normal. He was kept appropriately in the surgical intensive care unit for the first postoperative night. I was on call that night. My chief told me to make sure that he had a good "pulmonary toilet." In that era, the focus was on getting patients to cough. It was not yet appreciated that inspiratory effort was much more important than coughing. Patients were verbally encouraged to cough, and if they could not exert a good cough effort, we resorted to nasal tracheal suction. In retrospect, any salutary effect we would get from nasotracheal suctioning was more likely due to involuntarily encouraging inspiratory effort than removing secretions. I spent quite a long time with this patient trying to get him to cough, and I did resort, on multiple occasions, to employing nasotracheal suctioning. By the next morning, he seemed to be doing quite well. His breathing effort was normal, and he was comfortable. During the night, I obtained an arterial blood gas and his pO2 was 59 mmHg. When I presented his situation on morning rounds in front of the entire team, I was asked what his repeat arterial blood gas revealed. I replied that I had not drawn one because the results previously obtained were so very close to his preoperative levels. For the next what seemed like 10 min to me, but was probably shorter,

I received a lecture on how any pO2 less than 60 mmHg was a pre-arrest blood gas and that this patient's life was "hanging in the balance." The experience was humiliating. As I matured as a surgeon over the years, my own added experience reassured me that the patient had not been "pre-arrest" and my decision-making that evening was correct and did not call for public embarrassment.

When I think back to these first two chief residents, I think about how I observed them continuously and noted their very different styles of leadership. Not having had any leadership training at that time, my conclusions were very basic. My first chief resident impressed me with his compassion for his patients. I like the fact that he communicated in a consistent manner so that his words and body language were consistent. I could easily understand what was expected of me, and I could approach him with any questions without feeling fearful. On the other hand, I was not secure with him as a leader and felt that I could possibly be served up as a sacrificial lamb if one of his decisions was not perfect. I was disappointed that he did not assume ultimate responsibility for the poor outcome.

Raven and his associates, as cited above, would classify his use of power as positional: He was my day-to-day boss; he also had the power of the expert with a greater knowledge base than the rest of the team. General Hertling, as referenced in his book, might have commented on his behavior as inconsistently demonstrating character. My first chief resident had some admirable qualities such as compassion and gentleness and was an excellent communicator. Being a leader is not a "9–5 job" in the sense that demonstrating character is a 24-h responsibility with the team always watching and observing their leader. All his resident team members had their eyes on their chief resident continuously. Whether he was upset or gratified with a given action was noted. When he shirked his responsibilities for delaying the operation for complete small bowel obstruction, that was also noted.

My second chief resident instilled in his team a culture of discipline and high expectations for excellence. He "ruled" with an iron fist, wielding his "positional, expert, and informational power." This could also be described as autocratic, coercive power, or transactional. In the era when I trained, 22 interns competed for "survival" for appointment as chief resident. There were only eight chief residents per year. This was called a pyramidal program. A chief resident had a tremendous amount of coercive power over an intern. The chances of any intern securing a chief resident spot after a poor evaluation by a chief resident were very low indeed. In today's state of graduate medical education, we have rectangular programs. If there are eight chief resident slots, only eight categorical first-year resident positions are filled. There is less of an opportunity for one poor evaluation to have that kind of effect.

Teams led by transactional, positional leaders will always be limited to only modest success, and that will be difficult to sustain over the long run. Over the short run, particularly in an emergency situation or running a surgical care service for a month or two, this may be a successful style in terms of clinical outcomes. It does not reflect well on a training program or lead to a culture that will attract the best and the brightest surgical resident candidates. Public humiliation, a demonstration of power, has not proved to be an effective strategy for achieving long-term success.

There has in the past been little leadership training for the newly anointed surgical chief resident. For me, training in the late 1970s, there was none. I learned to do the surgical chief resident job by observing my previous chiefs and selecting the characteristics that I thought were worth emulating and rejecting the others.

As a general surgery chief resident, I was involved in a situation where one of the nurses missed an important written order. I had a conversation with her about the missed order, done in private, but did not pursue any further action. That nurse had otherwise been diligent in her care, and my patient ultimately did well. My chat with her pointed out the specific issue. I think I earned her loyalty by dealing with it one-on-one, in private, and not escalating my response. Afterward, I had the feeling that she looked out for my patients with a little extra effort. When I thought about how I handled that interaction, I was impressed by how well it worked out for my patients.

I came away from that one experience with a new (for me) effective leadership technique. It involved not being shy about pointing out what was not done optimally and doing it in private to avoid public humiliation. I named this my "squeeze and release" technique. In my mind, I thought of this as giving a "squeeze" of disapproval and then quickly put it in the past, the "release." It worked well over the years to improve outcomes and win respect. When I think about it today, I suspect I came off as someone who expected excellence but was not going to be abusive. Perhaps this created an environment for open communication without fear of retribution and embarrassment. On the other hand, I refused to tolerate repetition of the same mistake. That behavior resulted in a private, not pleasant conversation, and would result in an escalated response. In the case of surgical residents, I recorded it in my written evaluation. Today, I look at the approach that I developed as a chief resident as consistently demonstrating character that demanded excellence but also demonstrated compassion.

Leadership for Surgical Residents: Working in Multidisciplinary Teams

All surgical residents must function within multidisciplinary teams. Examples of these teams are trauma resuscitation or cardiac arrest and code response teams. I have observed these teams in action starting as a surgical resident participant, a team leader, and the one with the ultimate responsibility, the service chief. I have noticed that one type of interaction seemed to occur repeatedly. This was inappropriate and counterproductive behavior between peers with lasting downstream effects. It was not until I had my second turn as a Trauma Service Chief that I could appreciate and understand the interpersonal dynamics and could then develop an effective strategy to deal with it.

Here is a classic example of the way this counterproductive behavior is usually manifested. In its usual presentation, a patient is brought into the Trauma

Resuscitation Bay with multiple injuries, and the Trauma Team responds. The team follows the standard ABCs of trauma care. The airway was established, and the trauma team leader, a senior general surgery resident, noted that there were decreased breath sounds on the right side. Preparations were made to insert a chest tube as the chest X-ray had revealed a hemo-pneumothorax. There was also a right lower extremity open tibia and fibula fracture. The orthopedic residents were starting to irrigate the fracture site when the midlevel trauma resident greeted them with nasty, condescending instructions not to irrigate the fracture before the chest tube was inserted. Two weeks later, the general surgery trauma residents informed me how unresponsive the orthopedic residents had become in terms of timeliness of consultations and agreeing to take patients in transfer. My residents wanted me to deal with this by involving the Orthopedics Chair. Clearly, the dynamic of demeaning communication during the resuscitation had carried over to the personal interaction between service residents, days, and weeks later.

My strategy for dealing with this type of issue was to create a standing special multidisciplinary orthopedic/trauma resident meeting for those involved in caring for patients on the trauma service. The goal of this meeting was to open the lines of communication. The idea was to clear the air. In this case, it was to explain the importance of the priority of treating the pneumothorax before the fracture. Most important was to get all the residents to understand how their interpersonal interactions impacted on providing excellent care. I wanted the residents to understand the "downstream" effects of poor interactions and the failures when not communicating in a respectful manner with their colleagues.

Lessons Learned for Surgical Residents

1. Surgical residents should be introduced to the concepts of medical leadership early in their training. Instruction in leadership styles and power dynamics will be helpful to the developing leader. The concept of tailoring leadership style to the situation or situational management [1] has its place. The leader has an obligation to include the team in decision-making whenever possible as this has great educational value, creating buy-in to shared goals and the best outcomes for patient care. As I learned from Mr. Vince Joseph: "Until you become a leader it is about growing yourself, but once you become a leader it is about growing others on your team." There are times when the emergent situation will call for authoritarian/transactional leadership.

2. Residents should understand the importance that as a chief resident or leader, the team is always observing you and drawing conclusions about your character. They will hang on to your every word and nuance. Lack of support will be duly noted.

3. The dynamics of multispecialty team function need to be taught as well. In the current language of leadership training, functioning in multidisciplinary teams is an example of leading sideways. The key to successfully leading those on the

same level is to employ open, multidirectional respectful communication. It is important to understand that people have memories and that today's insulting behavior is tomorrow's bad clinical outcome.

Reference

1. Hersey P, Blanchard KH. Management of organizational behavior: utilizing human resources. Allendale: Prentice Hall; 1969.

Chapter 4
Operative Leadership for the Newly Minted Surgeon

After completing surgical residency and/or fellowship training, the new surgeon is faced with multiple challenges. He or she will be called on to lead the assigned Operating Room team. The circulator, scrub tech, or nurse, and the first assistant, whether it is a resident or registered nurse first assistant, and anesthesia team all will be looking to the attending surgeon to safely lead and navigate the operation. The operating room is one of the highest-stress areas of the hospital. If it is an elective operation, the patient, the patient's loved ones, and the surgical team are all expecting a perfect outcome. Any behaviors that will adversely affect achieving the optimal outcome will increase the stress in the operating room dramatically. The successful attending surgeon must master the art of projecting confidence without arrogance while allowing open lines of communication for all the team members. Failure to do this will inhibit optimal team performance to the detriment of the patient.

In the early 1990s, I was the Chief of the Trauma Service at one of the largest inner-city trauma centers in the country, the Kings County Hospital Center ("The County") in Brooklyn, New York. A brand new trauma attending reported for work after completing his fellowship at a prestigious, smoothly run, high volume, well-funded trauma center. His experience was mostly with blunt trauma patients. He was now working within a different culture with a preponderance of penetrating trauma. Although it had a glorious history, "The County" was a public city hospital that was not well funded and did not always function smoothly. We were still able to deliver excellent care and bring forth innovative advances in trauma care. This was accomplished mainly through the superhuman efforts of the dedicated medical and nursing staff.

I forewarned my new surgeon to expect great differences in our center from the one he had just left. As we debriefed after one of his first night call experiences, he complained bitterly about the inefficiencies of the OR team. He was concerned about how slowly they responded when passing instruments. After speaking with the nursing staff, it became obvious to me that as the case became more stressful,

S. Z. Trooskin, *An Introduction to Medical Leadership for Surgeons*, https://doi.org/10.1007/978-3-031-44264-3_4

this young surgeon exhibited more anxiety, frustration, anger, and rudeness in his dealings with the staff. As he continued to malign the staff, their performance deteriorated even further.

There have been studies that explore the relationship between leadership style in the operating room and team efficiency [1]: Transactional or dogmatic leadership ("do what I say now"), as opposed to transformational leadership (by inquiring "what is holding us back"), resulted in less efficient team functioning in the operating room. In short, the attending surgeon can make a stressful situation more stressful with their behavior or calm the seas and improve team function, dynamics, and efficiency. I had, very early on, come to the following conclusion: It is an absolute necessity for surgeons, as the leader, to develop techniques to control their own stress in order to best manage the team's stress. This is necessary for leading in the operating room and in leading the care of sick patients in the trauma resuscitation areas or intensive care units.

I do not recommend that surgeons take antianxiety medications to reduce their stress levels. They may dull the senses. How then can surgeons control their own behavior when unforeseen, stressful events come up during an operation?

Anxiety and stress reduction can be taught and learned. For me, the most effective stress reduction technique was preparation. An effective surgeon leader of the operative team should anticipate and consider the different scenarios of what could possibly go wrong and have a plan ready to deal with them. I found that preparing for the next few days calmed me down. As a resident, I would spend my downtime preparing for the next day by dealing with whatever issues were making me "nervous." As a PGY-3, I was assigned 5 months on the Trauma Service at Bellevue Hospital Center. As the senior resident on call, I knew that I would be leading the resuscitation and early management for patients coming in through door of the Emergency Department. During that every other night rotation (that was before the current work hour restrictions), I spent my free time reading about the management of every possible injury. It worked! My confidence grew as my knowledge base and experience increased. I had learned that if I knew how to recognize the circumstances that were making me anxious and knew what to do in the correct sequence, my anxiety miraculously decreased. I was in control!

As a new attending, I developed the habit of preparing for the week by reviewing my schedule during the prior weekend. I would prepare for my elective cases. I examined the patients' medical records to make sure that all the details were covered and that their preoperative evaluations had been completed. Did the cardiac stress test come back negative? Did I hear back from the cardiologist and the pulmonologist? What loose ends were pending? What were the potential pitfalls that I might face in the operating room? In this manner, I prepared for the week and was ready.

Nine years after completing my general surgical residency, I accepted the position of Chief of Trauma Surgery at the Kings County Medical Center. When I started at the very busy inner-city trauma center, "The County," I knew I would face many new challenges. At my previous institution, Robert Wood Johnson University Hospital, we took care of mostly patients suffering from blunt traumatic injuries

(95%). I had backup from board certified vascular and thoracic surgeons. I would identify the presence of those injuries, call the subspecialists, and the operative management would be done by those services. When I relocated to Brooklyn, I would have to manage, as the operating surgeon, major vascular and thoracic injuries. I had plenty of experience with these operations as a resident, but that had been more than 9 years in the past. The thought of again having that responsibility made me very anxious. I went to the literature and reviewed the essentials. I arranged some support with colleagues in those disciplines to help me if needed. The fact that I had someone to call if I needed help was quite comforting.

I had learned in my first few months, after completing my surgical residency, that there was no shame in calling for help in the operating room. I found that having a backup plan, which was to have an experienced surgeon available, also helped me to control my anxiety. I had, by the time I retired, performed approximately 6000 thyroid and parathyroid operations. That said, I did not start my career as an expert. The first thyroidectomy that I attempted as a new surgical attending at Robert Wood Johnson University Hospital started smoothly. After I finished mobilizing the first lobe, I realized that I could not identify the recurrent nerve. I kept at it to no avail and was concerned that I would injure that delicate structure. Instead of panicking or losing my cool, I called my senior-most associate. I had arranged for Dr. John Landor to be available if needed. I needed him. He came into the room, scrubbed up, and repositioned the retractor that I was using to get lateral traction on the strap muscles. That small adjustment of the lateral retraction was all it took for him to expose the location of the recurrent laryngeal nerve. He quickly spread tissue with a mosquito clamp, and there, almost like magic, appeared the recurrent nerve. I immediately realized my technical error was that as I had the medical student pull harder; I was, in effect, turning the head and neck toward him and away from me. I was moving the recurrent nerve progressively more lateral and posterior out of my view. I was very relieved to safely find the recurrent nerve without having injured it. Calling my senior colleague was helpful as I learned something, and the patient was spared a complication.

I was never embarrassed to ask for help. My primary concern was to take excellent care of the patient, and I lived by the Latin term *primum non nocere*, "first do no harm." If that required me getting help, so be it. I did not care if my team knew that I needed help. It was not a sign of weakness. Why? They observed that my most important concern was for the patient. That type of attitude and behavior helped to gain their respect. I knew that in and out of the operating room I had the reputation or label of being extremely demanding. I appreciated that my attention to detail sometimes may have made my operations tedious for my team, but they understood that the safety of our patients was my primary concern.

I learned to accept help from whatever the source. I remember one operation where the location of the enlarged parathyroid was not in the place identified by the preoperative studies, which by itself was not at all unusual. As I was dissecting in the superior mediastinum, the third-year medical student asked me about something he saw a little higher in the neck. I immediately stopped and asked him to point out to me exactly where he saw it. Lo and behold, he found the enlarged parathyroid! I was quite pleased and complimented him but was also gratified that I created an environment where a student would be comfortable speaking up. Finding the enlarged parathyroid was more important than who had found it. My favorite question for medical students in the operating room was to ask them to name the most important person in the room. Saying it was anyone but the patient was met with an explanation by me of why we were truly there.

I accepted help from any member of the team. It was one of the reasons I could not wait to have a consistent team to work with in the operating room. When I arrived back at Robert Wood Johnson University Hospital in 2002, I requested to be assigned my own team in the operating room. That request was not honored until I had a large, predictable operative volume. Although I was the new Surgical Service Chief, I had to be patient. My first consistent scrub tech understood the role I insisted that she play in my operating room. She had to be an active contributor. Given Tiffany's outgoing, vivacious personality, it was not a reach for her. Her first contribution was to suggest some different instruments that I might find useful. She introduced me to the insulated cautery tip, which just left 2 mm of exposed conducting metal. Since I was operating deep in the neck via small incisions doing thyroid and parathyroid operations, the insulated tip was a huge safety improvement. I did not spare the praise or encouragement for her future suggestions.

When Tiffany moved to Ohio, I interviewed candidates to replace her. The woman who was interested in being part of the team was very shy and quiet, and I stressed the importance of her being comfortable speaking her mind. I explained that one important aspect of her job would be to keep me "out of trouble." Cheryl never disappointed me. I was blessed to work in the operating room with people who tolerated my demanding style and were not intimidated in speaking their minds. I worked primarily with one circulating nurse over the last 15 years. Leigh was never afraid to speak up. If she thought I was doing something out of the usual format, she was not shy in asking what my intentions were. One day when I was about ready to break scrub, she asked: "Are you purposefully not transplanting the parathyroid tissue today? Don't you transplant it before you close the skin?" I had completely forgotten that I had the scrub tech hold on to parathyroid tissue that I wanted to autotransplant before closing the incision. Autotransplant of minced parathyroid tissue that had lost its blood supply is a method to prevent the long-term complication of low serum calcium. That was just one of many times Leigh had kept me out of trouble.

Lessons Learned for the Newly Minted Surgeon

1. Surgeons in the operating room are the de facto leaders of the OR team. As the one with the moral contract with the patient, the surgeon is ultimately responsible for the outcome. The new surgeon must learn to control his/her own anxiety to have an optimally functioning team. Public displays of anxiety with harsh, critical language lead to the deterioration of team function and are unfortunately

contagious. This type of transactional leadership style in the operating room has been shown to be counterproductive.

2. Techniques to lower surgeon anxiety include establishing a routine of preparation in advance of the operations. The surgeon should be prepared with "what if" strategies so that various "unexpected events" are anticipated. Arranging backup help to be available if needed can also be an anxiety-reducing strategy.

3. The surgeon establishes the culture in the operating room and is responsible for educating the operating team. Most importantly, the surgeon is the one person who can keep the lines of team communication open to the ultimate benefit of the patient.

4. Operations need to be conducted in an orderly sequence of steps with all team members knowledgeable in what comes next. It is the surgeon, as team the leader, who has the responsibility to ensure that the team is highly functioning. Working in a highly functioning team can be anxiety reducing for all team members. One measure of the team culture is to note if your team frequently asks questions.

Reference

1. Hu YY, Parker SH, Lipsitz SR, Arriaga AF, Peyre SE, Corso KA, Roth EM, Yule SJ, Greenberg CC. Surgeons' leadership styles and team behavior in the operating room. J Am Coll Surg. 2016;222(1):41–51.

Chapter 5
Using Emotional Intelligence to Grow Surgical Practice Referrals

Surgeons must be the leaders who grow their own clinical practices. What does it take to develop and lead a practice? When I was a surgical resident, I listened very carefully to my chairman, Dr. Frank Spencer, who had a lot of advice for his residents in developing a practice. He had a track record of success that made him credible. He had developed and was leading a large referral practice in cardiac surgery. His initial success was related to his surgical training at Johns Hopkins. That department literally made open heart surgery routine and achieved excellent outcomes.

The "Boss," as he was referred to, was very good at making his points by employing alliterations. He would say that the key to developing a practice is the 3 "A's": Affability, Availability, and Ability. The obvious interpretation: The surgeon looking to develop a practice needs to be affable or in other words approachable by referring physicians and patients. The surgeon should be available: If a doctor calls you, call back as soon as you can and get the patient into the office/clinic expeditiously. See that new consult as soon as possible. The last key is to be able, to be good at what you do and deliver excellent results consistently.

The "Boss" would also advise us that when dealing with someone who was angry and unreasonable, employ the use the 3 "L's": Listen, Laugh, and Leave. In short, do not make a public spectacle of the situation when you cannot possibly win. The laugh is more a smile or a head shake—do not lose your cool—and the leave refers to just politely walking away. Today's leadership courses would refer to the 3 "A's" and 3 "L's" as effectively leading sideways, leading your peers via your behavior.

As I prepared to start my clinical practice, that was the only advice that I had. Looking back 40-plus years later, it continues to be solid advice. An additional lesson that I picked up early as an attending surgeon was to treat everyone nicely. When you did not, people noticed. During my first few weeks after starting as a general surgeon attending Rutgers Medical School and Middlesex General Hospital (ultimately, both were renamed as Rutgers Robert Wood Johnson Medical School and Robert Wood Johnson University Hospital, respectively), I was asked by one of

S. Z. Trooskin, *An Introduction to Medical Leadership for Surgeons*, https://doi.org/10.1007/978-3-031-44264-3_5

the gastroenterologists to see a patient in the medical intensive care unit. The patient was having an active massive upper gastrointestinal bleed. I handled the situation the same way I had as a resident at Bellevue. I immediately took over the resuscitative efforts. The medical residents had inserted only a tiny "butterfly" intravenous catheter, and the surgical residents were struggling to insert the much-needed large-bore IV. Apparently, I was not very polite in my comments as I took over and inserted the intravenous catheter, completed the resuscitation, and took the patient expeditiously to the operating room, where we successfully controlled the bleeding from the gastroduodenal artery. I was very happy that the patient had an uneventful recovery. A few days later, the referring gastroenterologist sought me out with this message. Although he was very glad that the patient did well, he had to let me know that if I ever treated the medical residents with disrespect again, he would never send me another patient. I had clearly flunked the affable part of that situation. I took his feedback to heart. Over the years, I took care of a multitude of his patients, including his family members. I am forever grateful for his comments that day because it helped me change my behavior. I eventually answered the question "You can take the surgeon out of Bellevue, but can you take Bellevue out of the surgeon?" with "Yes, you can take Bellevue out of the surgeon."

Some of the lessons for surgeons leading in the operating room also apply to leading in the office or clinic. It is important to remember that the most important opinion regarding clinic efficiency and effective function is that of the patient. A successful office is one that is patient friendly. If the surgeon's goal is to follow the simple advice embodied in the "3 A's", then the office and everyone who works in that office must have buy-in for that same concept.

It is important to appreciate that patients approach their visit to the surgeon's office with a tremendous amount of anxiety. It is important to recognize this. If one steps into the patient's shoes, one can conclude that the visit is the most important thing the patient will do that day. This is particularly true with patients with cancer. I did not appreciate this until I was approached by a member of my own staff after she had an abnormal mammogram. I performed an operative needle localization and biopsy. (It was during the era before stereotactic biopsy availability.) That was followed by an axillary dissection and external beam radiation for a small invasive cancer. She did very well. I had expected that the initial treatment period would be quite traumatic for her. I noticed that she took her cues from me. She seemed to be comforted by my expressions of confidence that she was going to do well. I think my daily availability for support was a great advantage and helped her to cope with the situation. As I went on this journey with her, I noticed that she was able to compartmentalize the trauma of having breast cancer. I could understand that the operation of lumpectomy, axillary dissection, and radiation was a godsend for her, as she did not have the daily reminder of a body deforming mastectomy. Over the years, I could see her anxiety increase in the days before her follow-up mammograms and office visits, and I would watch that anxiety rapidly dissipate with the information that there was no evidence of cancer.

In my own family, I could sense the anxiety that was associated with getting a screening mammogram. There is only one reason to have a mammogram: It is to answer the question, "Do I have cancer?" Patients want to get those results as soon as possible, and everyone interacting with the patient needs to understand this. This feeling of dread that patients experience while waiting for test results is not confined to mammograms. I saw it daily with my patients undergoing thyroid ultrasounds or thyroid mapping studies for preoperative evaluation for the involvement of lymph nodes in the lateral neck or in the yearly follow-up studies. It was clear to me that the takeaway message was that all my patients were anxious, brought on by antici-pating what I was going to do or say.

Today, patients have ready access to their electronic medical records and can check the results themselves. Although easy access to results may sound like a theo-retical advantage, it also holds the potential to heighten patient anxiety as results are frequently reported in the technical language of the specialist. Laboratory results are quantitative, and those results can also lead to confusion for the layperson. A patient can get concerned about a slightly low or elevated MCV on the CBC but have a normal hemoglobin and hematocrit. They do not know that they are looking at an inconsequential abnormal result. Medical offices can feel overwhelmed by patient inquiries about results. The office staff must understand that there are issues of workflow and there are the patient's concerns about their mortality. I was reminded of this conflict of staff vs. patient priorities at almost every office session. I fre-quently fell behind in my schedule when seeing patients, as I tried to spend enough time to meet patient needs and reduce their anxiety. The nursing staff would tell me about the complaints actively being received by the front desk. I noticed that the patients' attitudes almost always improved after getting into the exam rooms and having "face time" with me. It was especially true after they had received good results. Patients generally will get angry if other patients need extra time with me and they must wait longer to see me. They also do not care if I am not feeling well that day because I have a boil on my butt. They are concerned about their mortality, and that needs to be recognized by the entire office team. In both the operating room and the clinic, the patient is the most important person in the room.

I readily admit that I have never had the joy of working in a superbly efficient office setting, with enough staff that was consistently happy. It therefore begged the question: If most practices do not have the resources to have a smooth, efficient office or clinic, how can the surgeon leader keep patients and staff as happy as pos-sible? It can be challenging, and I do not have the perfect answer. One answer goes back to the basics of culture, character, and the application of compassion. The surgeon must demonstrate excellence of character and try to create a culture that respects the needs of the patient and the staff. If the surgeon behaves in a manner that understands the needs of the patient, the staff will notice and change their behavior to be consistent with the surgeon leader. If they cannot adapt, they will need to find another place to work with a less demanding surgeon.

As part of a multispecialty medical school practice, I frequently did not have the opportunity to add staff or have as much influence on clinic function as I would have liked. I therefore attempted to control what I could. Personally, I could try to set a good example by being as patient friendly as possible. I tried to always do the basics and teach the medical students and surgical residents those basics. The basics are to knock on a door before entering, say hello and introduce yourself to new patients; if you know the patient well, make a comment or question that demonstrates that you remember them. Always sit down and make eye contact. It can be challenging to make enough eye contact when you have the electronic medical record on the screen between you and the patient.

I found that patients accepted that I needed to look at the screen if I prefaced the screen look with comments such as "Let me refresh my memory" or "Let's review your tests results together." I frequently would look at the actual radiographic studies at that time and show them the findings on the screen. My aim was to involve them in what I was doing. At the end of the visit, I would summarize the plan for the patient. For follow-up visits, I liked to dictate my notes in front of the patient and invite them to correct me if I was not accurate. Listening to my dictation was a good way to reinforce the plan of care for the patient.

When I started my first position after residency, I noted that the practice had the surgical residents on call take all the night inquiries from the patients. The patients were advised to call the hospital operators with any questions that may arise after the office closed and ask to speak with the resident on call. After a few weeks of clinical activity, I realized that the residents were not equipped to deal with outpatient issues as they arose in real time. Most of their time on call was spent working up new admissions, dealing with critical issues, and scrubbing in on emergency operations. They also lacked the experience and in some cases the judgement to deal with the outpatient problems. My patients were not happy about my lack of availability. It took a while, but I eventually convinced my division chief to employ an answering service. I did not realize it at the time, but I was practicing "leading up" effectively.

Over the years, I developed an appreciation of Dr. Spenser's "3 A's" advice of being available, affable, and able. The "able" part became one of the finer points of practice building. It translated into being able to do operations that others could not do and getting great results. More on that will be presented below. In addition to getting great results, the surgeon needs to build a highly skilled and functioning multidisciplinary team and continue to develop excellent relationships with referring docs, making sure they receive important follow-up information. Make sure that your patients feel well taken care of by being "available," by educating them and their families. These days "warm and fuzzy" continues to go a long way with patients.

There was a time in history when "warm and fuzzy," respectful communication skills or emotional intelligence were not the primary requirements for practice building. Historically, achieving excellent results while performing the most advanced, modern techniques, and being one of only a few surgeons who could accomplish this was more than enough. In previous eras, affability and availability were not as important as being that special surgeon who could attract a large patient base via the safe application of the latest technology. Hospital and clinical administrative leaders would tolerate untold amounts of "bad behavior" if the surgeon could put "butts in beds." A perfect example of this was William Stewart Halsted, generally considered the "Father of American Surgery." In the late nineteenth and early twentieth centuries, he made innumerable protean contributions to surgical education, operative techniques, and most importantly created a school of surgery at Johns Hopkins whose focus was on making operations routinely safe. I would suggest reading some of his papers and his biography [1, 2]. The fact is, he made operations such as hernia repair, operative treatments for breast cancer, and thyroid operations routinely safe by carefully analyzing his results and involving his patients' feedback. In that respect, he was a terrific role model. His resident trainees were in great demand and were recruited as chairmen by the major medical school hospitals because of the outstanding results they could consistently obtain.

The great Dr. Halsted was also flawed as a person and a leader. He was a stern taskmaster with a dour personality. Although he had established the surgical residency training system that was widely imitated, he was also very autocratic in that residents could not complete their training until Dr. Halsted thought they were ready. It did not matter how many years it took until the man was convinced that the resident was ready. Dr. Halsted had a major personal problem that was widely known by his peers and superiors: For most of his long and successful career, Dr. Halsted was a narcotic addict!

It was thought that his pioneering work introducing the use of local anesthetic into surgical practice led to his addiction. He experimented on himself utilizing first saline injections and later cocaine injected into the skin. Cocaine is a very effective local anesthetic and has a chemical structure very similar to modern non-addicting local anesthetic agents such as lidocaine. His landmark paper on the use of cocaine as an effective local anesthetic seems to have been authored while he was under the influence of cocaine. The style exhibited in that paper was replete with run-on sentences and was very different from the concise nature of his previous and subsequent papers. His cocaine addiction was treated by giving him morphia. His well-known career-long addiction to morphia was mostly overlooked by his peers. His sometimes long absences from the hospital were well-documented in the minutes of the Executive Medical Board of the Johns Hopkins Hospital. In today's lexicon, he was enabled by his physicians and superiors. I am sure his clinical and educational successes, which delivered patients and prestige to the institution, led to the "forgiveness of his numerous sins." This behavior obviously would not be tolerated today. Success today requires much more than great outcomes, and most medical staff bylaws have a zero-tolerance policy not only for alcohol and drug use but also for bad behavior that creates a hostile work environment. Twenty years ago, if a surgeon had a large practice and got great results or did cutting-edge procedures, bad behavior might have been overlooked. Loud, abusive behavior such as throwing instruments was frequently tolerated. It is no longer tolerated, and behavior like that will quickly get out into the public realm, defeating attempts to build a practice. Bad behavior will also most likely get the surgeon invited to appear in front of the Medical Executive Committee to face potential disciplinary actions.

Mastering cutting-edge techniques is an excellent strategy for practice building. It must be kept in mind that today's cutting-edge technical advances will have a shelf life that is finite. The development of open-heart surgery is one remarkable example of cutting edge that has become passe over time. It is worth studying in terms of practice building. Cardiopulmonary bypass was necessary to enable successful open-heart surgery. Although numerous institutions were trying to develop a successful working model, Dr. John Gibbon at Jefferson Medical College in Philadelphia did the first human operation in 1952 using cardiopulmonary bypass [3]. Nonetheless, it was the group at Hopkins that worked out the details to make the operations safe.

Halsted's successor as chairman of the department, Alfred Blalock, had attracted and recruited an outstanding group of surgical residents. Under his guidance, in the classic Hopkins tradition, this group made the use of cardiopulmonary bypass and cardiac surgery a safe and routine operation. By the mid-1960s, each of these young cardiac surgeons was recruited to other institutions to develop cardiac surgery programs. Dr. David Sabiston went to Duke University, Henry T. Bahnson was recruited to the University of Pittsburgh, Dr. John Kirkland to Alabama, and Dr. Frank Spencer came to New York University.

They were attracted by offers to become department chairs and the potential to be well-remunerated for their services. Each of these individuals developed highly successful programs. Patients traveled great distances to have their open-heart surgery performed by a Hopkins-trained cardiac surgeon. To handle the ever-increasing volume of patients that were referred to them in short order, the cardiac surgeons developed fellowship training programs in cardiothoracic surgery. The result of creating numerous fellowship training programs was to increase the number of surgeons who were experts at these operations. The best and brightest of the fellows initially stayed at the parent institution to work with their mentors. Over the years, as the number of cardiac surgery fellowship trained surgeons increased, more surgeons were available to be recruited to other university hospitals. These institutions wanted to keep these well-reimbursing patients in their home institutions, and patients were happy to get their care close to home.

Therefore, these former fellows were highly sought after and recruited to develop new cardiac surgery programs. In those early years, the focus was on institutions increasing patient volume as the care of cardiac patients was well-remunerated. Cardiac surgeons who could do the operations expeditiously and obtain good results rapidly built more high-volume programs. There was little scrutiny of their behavior if the program grew successfully. Surgeon behavior, good or bad, no matter how ugly, was tolerated. Cardiologists had little choice but to refer to local cardiac surgeons if they wanted to continue to be involved in their own patients' care through the perioperative period. As more and more fellowship training programs were established in the following two to three decades, the paradigm shifted. The cardiac surgeons gradually began to lose control of the programs to cardiologists, hospitals, and hospital systems. There was literally a glut of highly skilled cardiac surgeons to choose from. Some cardiology groups hired their own surgeons and retained total control of their patients. If the cardiologists did not "enjoy working" with a particular surgeon, that surgeon could easily be replaced with one who was better behaved or more compliant. In general, it became much easier to begin to treat the surgeons as technicians. Since access to patients was now controlled by cardiologists, they were the ones with great influence in their home institutions. In the 1990s, in a city like Philadelphia, cardiologists were successful at moving their large practice from one institution to another and by offering their volume and obtaining in return via legal monetary perks (within the Stark Regulations, i.e., by obtaining directorships and other types of administrative roles) or by becoming highly paid employees of hospital systems.

The phenomenon of the success achieved by early adopters in practice building, followed by the development of highly trained competitors and the loss of patient control, has been repeated in just about every discipline in medicine. It was seen in the introduction of coronary angioplasty and later coronary stent placement for interventional cardiologists. Interventional radiologists and vascular surgeons also have experienced similar potential to lose patient control.

Today's young surgeons must understand this trend and learn how to deal with it. It is important to look into the future, for both the near and the long term. The newly minted surgeon needs to decide which techniques and procedures are currently worthy of early adoption and which may become routine in the future. The lifespan of these new techniques needs to be determined. Surgeons should understand that they may need to reinvent themselves and be ready to be early adopters at multiple points if they are going to have a long successful career and maintain as much control of their patients as possible. Yes, there is hope, and it can be done successfully in the current era where patients are routinely referred by a primary care doctor or a medical specialist.

I gleaned several lessons from observing the early experience around the introduction of laparoscopic cholecystectomy. The laparoscopic approach to general surgery operations started in the late 1980s and clearly represented the future of many procedures. It offered less pain, more rapid recovery, shorter hospital stays, and earlier return to daily life and work, as well as better cosmetic results. At most hospitals, the blueprint for introducing this procedure was for the surgeon to take a didactic course and practice on a few pigs, and the surgeon was then declared ready to do this procedure on patients! What we saw, in addition to the benefits of the operation, was a very large increase in bile duct injuries [4].

Early adopters of laparoscopic cholecystectomy saw a very rapid and large growth in surgical referrals. Over the next decade, the procedure became safer and was part of the armamentarium of all general surgeons. In the initial introductory phase, some general surgeons actively chose not to learn the new technique. They did not believe that laparoscopic surgery was a great advance, was too dangerous, or they were just too set in their ways to learn the procedure. They then experienced their referral base drying up! The lesson to be learned here is obvious.

There are some more subtle lessons, not generally appreciated, that are important for the young surgeon seeking to develop a successful, high-volume practice. Some of these I learned by studying successful surgeons. In Philadelphia, I was quite fortunate to work closely with a wonderful vascular surgeon. We shared clinic time, and I had the opportunity to observe how Dr. Andrew Roberts ran his practice. Dr. Roberts always acted like a gentleman and always treated his team and patients well with respect and kindness. He saw patients all day on Tuesdays and Thursdays. He made sure a lunch break for his team was scheduled for the day's work. The entire team, as a group, would head to the cafeteria for lunch. This highly functioning team figuratively "whistled why they worked," and I could tell that they really enjoyed coming to work every day and were proud of the way they cared for patients.

I also noted that Andy did very few emergency vascular operations for patients cared for in his outpatient practice. Previously, I had witnessed the patients of other vascular surgeons calling the office or more frequently presenting to the Emergency Department with sudden onset of peripheral extremity ischemia. That rarely occurred in Andy's practice, as he monitored his patients at frequent intervals with noninvasive testing. As the monitored blood flow deteriorated from intimal hyperplasia or disease progression, he would do an angiogram and intervene before the development of the ischemic emergency with either a scheduled angioplasty or operation.

I appreciated that by monitoring his patients closely at scheduled intervals, he ultimately improved his patients' care. He maintained control over his patients and did not outsource this to the patient's primary care physicians or cardiologists, who may not be sensitive to the subtle signs of decreased peripheral blood flow. He was not dependent on those other physicians sending the patients back to him when the threats of tissue loss, amputation, or infection had increased. There is a benefit to both the patient and the surgeon to follow patients with chronic diseases long term.

As I made the transition from being a general surgeon with subspecialty expertise in trauma and surgical critical care to a thyroid/parathyroid surgeon, I borrowed shamelessly from my vascular colleague. As I developed my new practice, I decided I would learn to do my own ultrasound-guided thyroid nodule biopsies. I would also "mother hen" my patients and spend the time and effort to follow my patients longitudinally. Not all specialties lend themselves to long-term surgical follow-up, but my patients certainly did. Patients with thyroid nodules are at risk for nodule growth. It became my practice to see patients with benign biopsies at appropriate intervals and monitor them for nodule growth. Fine needle biopsies of thyroid nodules also have a significant incidence of false negative biopsies. I made sure that those patients understood that phenomenon and returned for a repeat biopsy to decrease the phenomenon of sampling error of one benign biopsy.

Patients with papillary thyroid cancer, as a group, have a 20% chance of having residual disease and needing more surgery in the future. I educated my patients about this risk and the need for close follow-up. I scheduled routine long-term follow-up visits with me, as I was the only individual who "knew the inside of their necks." After the postoperative period, I would make sure the patient was seen by either me or the endocrinologist at 6-month intervals. At a minimum, I would see the patient with thyroid cancer yearly and make sure they were monitored by me and or the endocrinologist at 6-month intervals. At those visits, the tumor markers and TSH suppression would be monitored, and physical examinations would be performed. I would make sure that the yearly ultrasound was ordered and results reviewed. My patients remarked that they felt comforted by my attention to detail and the possibility of identifying residual cancer as early as possible.

Primary hyperparathyroidism used to be thought to be cured by removing the adenoma(s) in almost every patient. The current data suggests [5] that the chance of developing another large gland is closer to 8% during the 10-year period following a successful neck exploration. As an early adopter of a directed operative approach in patients diagnosed with primary hyperparathyroidism by utilizing a rapid intra-operative hormone assay, I had always followed my postop patients very closely. I wanted to treat secondary hyperparathyroidism, which I noted in almost a third of my patients in the postoperative period. I monitored and treated my patient's vitamin D deficiency aggressively as a certain percentage were predisposed to recurrence. I kept my patients well-informed of the need for closer monitoring; if the patients did develop another large gland, they would not be surprised and would return to me for treatment.

I was also an early adopter of performing outpatient thyroid and parathyroid operations and the performance of the procedure using local anesthesia (superficial cervical block) to be able to offer these awake procedures selectively. The techniques of employing local anesthesia and same-day discharge had been described by Paul LoGerfo et al. [6] in publications that had a significant number of patients. I initially did these operations successfully in low volume while in Philadelphia without a lot of fanfare or comments from colleagues. After I was recruited back to Robert Wood Johnson Medical School and Robert Wood Johnson University Hospital, my new colleagues were quite vocal in declaring that what I was doing was dangerous, that patients would lose their airway at home, die, and that I would be sued and ruined! None of the above happened. Our excellent results were presented at a national meeting and subsequently published [7]. My ability to selectively send patients home after 6 h of observation turned out to be successful. There was no doubt that offering this type of cutting-edge care enhanced my referral base.

Another lesson for creating a successful program is to surround yourself with multidisciplinary experts. I built an operating room team that included an interested anesthesiologist, who quickly became adept at dealing with difficult airways. I would send complex patients to her for preoperative evaluation. She collaborated with me on refining and perfecting patient selection for the performance of thyroidectomy and neck exploration for patients with primary hyperparathyroidism under local anesthesia. We continually finely tuned our system so it could routinely function smoothly. I involved the Post Anesthetic Recovery Room nursing staff in monitoring patients and designing the protocol for postoperative evaluation. No patient was discharged at 6 h without me personally examining the patient. Most importantly, I ensured that I would be immediately available to my team and the patients.

I realized that a well-organized practice needed to be established to effectively handle the increased volume. I stressed to my team the importance of focusing on patient satisfaction. To make sure that patients felt that "warm and fuzzy" feeling, I worked to improve patient education. We purchased the Thyroid Book [8], a third-party publication, to give each patient with a thyroid problem. I prepared handouts on thyroid and parathyroid anatomy, physiology, operations, and complications for thyroid and parathyroid operations. I did not spare the details. I explained graphically, using hand drawn illustrations (the quality of those was not anything to brag about) that included the parathyroid glands, superior and recurrent nerves, and where a tracheostomy would be placed if needed. I made templates for my dictations so that I could document that I had personally obtained the informed consent and discussed the potential complications in detail.

As my practice grew rapidly, I found that it was difficult to do a comprehensive presentation to individual patients and continue to effectively manage the ever-increasing volume of new patients. I was seeing approximately 10–15 new patients a week and operating on about 10 a week. I decided to initiate educational sessions for new patients and their families prior to the initial visit with me. My staff, on scheduling the first visit, notified the patients that we would meet in a classroom, that it would be HIPPA compliant, and that no one should reveal personal information. They were informed that attendance was mandatory and that they had to be prepared to spend most of the morning in the office. Initially, I purposefully made these presentations very low-tech, using color markers and a whiteboard. I wanted the lights on and to retain the ability to interact with the patients. I could therefore make eye contact and answer questions in real time. I was somewhat surprised that the patients and I bonded during these sessions. During the COVID pandemic, when we could not congregate in a classroom, I prepared a YouTube video that the new patients were required to see prior to the initial visit. When comparing the two methods of imparting information to patients, I concluded that each method had different advantages. The obvious advantage of the classroom was that I could have personal interactions with the patients while I answered their questions. These sessions were quite long (about 2 h) and therefore more labor intense on my part. The video was more professional and allowed the patients to refer repeatedly to parts that they did not understand. It was impossible to get every patient to look at the video prior to their appointment, and these patients subsequently required more in-office time. On balance, in retrospect, the low-tech approach seemed to be the better method for departing the necessary information.

To compensate for the many inefficiencies in my outpatient clinic that I could not control, I had to employ several workarounds. I made sure that every patient that I operated on over the last 20 years had my cell phone number. The night before the operation, I called every patient to touch base and answer any questions. Prior to the operation, usually on the morning of the operation, I reviewed their postoperative instructions in detail and when to call for swelling and paresthesia. They were specifically told that if they did develop breathing issues, they were instructed to go to the nearest emergency department immediately. I made sure that they went home with written instructions even before this was made standard hospital practice.

Lessons Learned for Referral Building

1. There is a very old lesson that the key to building a successful practice is to follow the "3 A's" of Availability, Affability, and Ability. This is now termed as demonstrating character and emotional intelligence when dealing with patients and colleagues.

2. As stressed previously, the surgeon's behavior in and out of the operating room and clinic is under almost continuous observation. Demonstrating honesty, character and emotional intelligence is critical to developing and maintaining a rich surgical referral base. Dressing down or insulting behavior while delivering needed care affects referrals. It is better to Listen, Laugh, and Leave, the "3 L's."
3. Patients seeking medical care appreciate recognition of their anxiety and vulnerability. "Warm and fuzzy" office staff behaviors go a long way to aiding patient satisfaction and word-of-mouth reputation building. Creating that kind of culture in the clinic is important. There are numerous low-cost, simple ways to accomplish this.
4. In the distant past, failure to consistently demonstrate professionalism would be tolerated if the practitioner had a robust practice that contributed mightily to the institution's "bottom line." That no longer holds true, and consistent bad behavior can result in dismissal from the medical staff.
5. It is important to understand the life cycle of early adoption of new technology. Some applications of new technology are nonstarters and not worth the investment. Others are game changers and to miss out will shrink the referral base (e.g., laparoscopy). Today's revolutionary advances are tomorrow's routine procedures (e.g., open heart surgery).
6. Long-term follow-up by the surgeon of chronic conditions like peripheral vascular disease or thyroid cancer is representative of excellent care as well as practice building and maintenance.

References

1. Halsted WS. Practical comments on the use and abuse of cocaine; suggested by its invariable successful employment in more than a thousand minor surgical operations. N Y Med J. 1885;xlii:294–5.
2. Imber G. Genius on the edge: the bizarre double life of Dr. William Stewart Halsted. New York: Kaplan; 2011.
3. Lena T, Amabile A, Morrison A, Torregrossa G, Geirsson A, Tesler UF, John H. Gibbon and the development of the heart-lung machine: the beginnings of open cardiac surgery. J Card Surg. 2022;37(12):4199–201.
4. Macintyre IM, Wilson RG. Laparoscopic cholecystectomy. BMJ. 1992;304(6829):777.
5. Szabo Yamashita T, Mirande M, Huang CT, Kearns A, Fyffe-Freil R, Singh R, Foster T, Thompson G, Lyden M, McKenzie T, Wermers RA, Dy B. Persistence and recurrence of hypercalcemia after parathyroidectomy over 5 decades (1965-2010) in a community-based cohort. Ann Surg. 2023;278(2):e309–13.
6. Spanknebel K, Chabot JA, DiGiorgi M, Cheung K, Curty J, Allendorf J, LoGerfo P. Thyroidectomy using monitored local or conventional general anesthesia: an analysis of outpatient surgery, outcome and cost in 1,194 consecutive cases. World J Surg. 2006;30(5):813–24.
7. Narayanan S, Arumugam D, Mennona S, Wang M, Davidov T, Trooskin SZ. An evaluation of postoperative complications and cost after short-stay thyroid operations. Ann Surg Oncol. 2016;23(5):1440–5.
8. Krames. The thyroid book: medical and surgical treatment of thyroid problems. Yardley: Krames; 2021.

Chapter 6
Participating Successfully in Hospital Committees

The key to functioning successfully within and then leading a committee is to understand the dynamics of members of the committee. There are important issues that one must understand, such as: What are the turfs that various members think they must protect? Can you build consensus, and are you ready to make compromises to make progress on your issue? Here are some lessons that I learned over the years.

In 1980, as a newly minted attending general surgeon, my chairman decided that I should serve on the Emergency Department and Critical Care Committees of the hospital. He thought that would fit nicely with my interests in Trauma and Surgical Critical Care. My first encounter with a hospital committee involved my concerns about delays in surgical involvement in patients presenting with massive gastrointestinal bleeding. My immediate thought was to bring this up at the very next Emergency Department Committee. My solution: All unassigned patients presenting to the hospital with GI bleeding should be admitted to the Surgical Services. I had a preliminary discussion with my chairman before the meeting, and then as part of new business, I brought it up at the committee. After minimal discussion, the matter quickly went to a vote. My vote was the only one in favor. My chairman was not surprised by the results. I suspected later that he wanted me to undergo the experience of learning firsthand how a committee functions.

As I analyzed the experience, I came to understand that there were issues related to potential referral patterns, remuneration, and residency training considerations that I had failed to appreciate. I learned the hard way that it was not smart to "spring" a new provocative idea on the committee without doing my homework. I should have canvased members of the group in advance of the meeting and put together a long-term strategy. It would have been more helpful, as a first step, to introduce the topic and listen to an open discussion by the group. Involving the entire group in developing a solution would have been more productive. In today's understanding of leadership styles and techniques, I should have been better at leading both sideways and leading up.

© The Author(s), under exclusive license to Springer Nature Switzerland AG 2023
S. Z. Trooskin, *An Introduction to Medical Leadership for Surgeons*, https://doi.org/10.1007/978-3-031-44264-3_6

Lesson Learned about Functioning in Committees

1. An experienced leader understands the dynamics and long-term effects of proposals and refrains from springing a new idea in the group.
2. Time spent listening to the members is time well spent. Understanding the different concerns and potential areas of agreements and disagreements as well as the willingness to compromise will prove to be very helpful.

Chapter 7
Leading/Starting a New Program

Building a new program from the ground up can be challenging for the most experienced leader. A lot of work needs to be done, and numerous potential pitfalls await. It is a formidable task. For example, a team on the ground needs to be built from the present talent and will also likely need to be buffeted by recruits from the outside. Multiple specialties must buy into the concept and supply support during the actual creation. It is important to have the leader's superiors on board with every planned step. It is critical for the medical leader to understand where this program is situated on the institution's overall priority list.

My first efforts to build a new program had an atypical beginning. The typical beginning for a new program starts with the institutional commitment and then the recruitment of the new leader. My first trial-and-error experience with building a new program began very differently. It started with an early observation, as a new member of the faculty, that the treatment of the trauma patients at my hospital was not optimal. In 1980, as a new junior faculty member, I witnessed the presentation of case of an injured elderly woman at a M&M Conference. I could not help but draw the conclusion that the care of the acutely injured was very disorganized.

At that time, there were two state designated demonstration project Level 1 Trauma Centers in the state of New Jersey. They were placed in the highly functioning existing trauma programs. One, located in Newark at New Jersey Medical School, had a lot of experience in treating the victims of penetrating trauma. The second was at Cooper Hospital in Camden, which had invested in developing a Trauma Center modeled on the Shock Trauma Unit at the University of Maryland. The call for demonstration projects initially went out from the state Office of Emergency Medical Services (OEMS) in an announcement in 1977. Both of those institutions completed the Request for Proposal (RFP). The response from UMD Robert Wood Johnson Medical School was one of ignoring the RFP. Three years later when I joined the department, I discovered that I was the only faculty member with any extensive experience in trauma care.

S. Z. Trooskin, *An Introduction to Medical Leadership for Surgeons*,
https://doi.org/10.1007/978-3-031-44264-3_7

My interest in developing a trauma program originated from my intense experience at Bellevue Hospital Medical Center as a surgical resident and my newfound concerns about the quality of care that I witnessed at my new hospital. The good news was that the nascent university hospital in New Brunswick had most of the pieces for optimal management of the acutely injured as described by the American College of Surgeons Committee on Trauma. That organization's literature [1] and members helped guide me through the process of improving the outcomes for trauma patients. I could and did shamelessly borrow from that detailed playbook and my much more experienced national colleagues. The bad news was that there were no systemic efforts to care for the acutely injured. In the beginning, I had no resources and no budget.

I started with the basics. We needed a well-equipped resuscitation area. My first effort was to take the top two nursing leaders in the Emergency Department on a field trip to Bellevue so I could show them the trauma resuscitation area and how the equipment was arranged around the stretcher. I gave them a list of all the necessary equipment needed for resuscitation. These ladies were kind enough to order a large Rubbermaid cart, which was delivered about a month later. Unfortunately, the equipment sat haphazardly unopened on the cart for weeks until my secretary and I, armed with a label maker, organized the cart and made it usable. The immediate availability of the equipment was an early success, a visible piece of evidence that helped the resuscitation efforts.

It was a time of challenging circumstances. In 1980, the hospital was 3 years into the affiliation agreement with the medical school to transform it from a struggling community hospital to the primary teaching affiliate of the medical school. Large investments were made in the new cardiac surgery program, the new surgical intensive care unit, the pediatric intensive care unit, and the renal dialysis program. All the necessary subspecialists were on the staff to qualify the hospital as a trauma center. The affiliation with the Rutgers Medical School added the potential for research in trauma care, and I therefore felt, if all the pieces could be put together, the qualifications for Level 1 Trauma Center could be met. I created a priority list: first, improve the quality of trauma care; second, convince both the hospital and the medical school that they should want to have a Level 1 Trauma Center. I had almost unilaterally decided that it was important for the citizens in central New Jersey, the hospital, and the medical school to have a Level 1 Trauma Center. No one gave me the assignment, but I nonetheless naively made it my passion and mission.

The leadership issues that I faced were protean. I had to build a team of individuals who could help me manage all the individual projects that would improve the quality of care. I had to convince my peers in the surgery department and in other departments that it was in their best interests to have a designated Level 1 Trauma Center. I had to cajole the Emergency Medical Technicians (EMTs) and paramedics to bring us the patients instead of the nearest hospital. I had to persuade the hospital that both the publicity of having the trauma center and attracting additional patients would be advantageous, not just as a "halo effect" but financially. The most difficult task was to deal with the "politics" of the university. The jewel of the campus in Newark was the Trauma Center, and the university wanted to expand the catchment area for it to include the blunt trauma victims from as much of the northern and central parts of the state as possible.

My chairman was skeptical about building a trauma program at that point in time, but he saw the potential benefits to the department, the school, and the hospital, giving me the approval to proceed. I do not think he anticipated the downstream headaches I would send his way. Here is just one small example. The Chair of Surgery at the time was a cardiothoracic surgeon, and the standard practice prior to my arrival was to call a thoracic surgery consultant to insert a chest tube. When I changed the protocol to have the trauma resuscitation team of general surgeons and their residents insert the chest tube in the Emergency Department without seeking a consult, the other thoracic surgeons were not happy. That action, as well as others over the succeeding months, netted me a visit to the chairman's office for discussions. I "survived" those meetings because there was no denying the need to do the best for the patients. He understood the importance of treating pneumothorax and hemothorax ASAP. I did agree to consult the thoracic surgeons after the chest tube went in, but the thoracic surgeons quickly tired of ex post facto consultations, and the practice stopped. It turned out there were many of those subsequent chairman meeting invitations for similar issues of disrupting the status quo.

In the early 1980s, I had no experience in leading the development of any program. There were no pertinent leadership courses that I knew about at the time, and no one suggested that I look for one. I had the experience of being a good surgeon: taking pride in delivering what I thought was the best surgical care for my patients; asking for help when I needed it; and when I failed, analyzing what went wrong, learning from it, and doing it differently next the time. I did have supportive mentors around me. The General Surgery Division Chief was onboard and very supportive. It took a while, but a Section of Trauma and Surgical Critical Care within the Division of General Surgery was created, and I was named the chief. The former Chief of Trauma in Newark, Dr. Ken Swan, was always available for any clinical questions that came up. Administratively, I was basically on my own with trial and error.

Building a group to help with clinical projects was not difficult. Over a relatively short time, a group of nurses from the operating room and the emergency department became true believers, as did the surgical residents. The paramedics came on board early as well. The hospital hosted the regional EMS communication center. New Jersey had a voluntary ambulance service staffed by volunteer EMTs and hospital-based paramedic units that would accompany the ambulances. How did I get the support of nurses and the pre-hospital providers? I used the formula that worked for many groups that I attempted to lead. I tried to be the nice, approachable surgeon, who listened to their concerns and recommendations. I took advantage of their desire and need to be educated in trauma care. For the nurses, I led small group discussions and gave lectures freely; for the paramedics, I provided medical leadership for their Pre-Hospital Trauma Life Support (PHTLS) courses and medical leadership for the University of Medicine and Dentistry School of Allied Health Professions. I became the medical director for their paramedic training course. In retrospect, these purely voluntary efforts, although time consuming, particularly because I did them on nights and weekends, were key to creating a dedicated loyal team. The pride engendered by the goal, by being part of the struggle to obtain the Level 1 designation and the visible proof of improved care, was a priceless recruiting tool.

I had to convince the other surgeons to participate willingly. The medical staff consisted of providers who were both full-time faculty and those in private practice. There were concerns regarding the potential loss of clinical income by the latter. I presented data on the effectiveness of trauma centers in reducing preventable deaths. I attempted to demonstrate fairness by rigidly following the ACS COT guidelines for trauma center designation. In other words, I borrowed from the national standards for excellence. I opened the trauma on-call schedule to all general surgeons provided they satisfactorily completed the ATLS Course and made themselves immediately available with no commitments at other hospitals while taking trauma calls. By playing my cards face-up and strictly following the ACS COT Guidelines for Trauma Center designation, I like to think I proved that I could be trusted to be an honest broker. My biggest support on the medical staff came from those in private practice, the Chief of the Division of Orthopedic Surgery, and two neurosurgeons. One of the neurosurgeons was a chief resident at NYU when I was an intern. Those gentlemen understood that ultimately getting a Level 1 Trauma Center designation would improve patient safety and increase patient volume.

I realized that the biggest challenge was convincing the leadership at the university that there should be a Level 1 Trauma Center for Central New Jersey. The next greatest challenge was to convince the hospital that a Trauma Center was something that they should need and want. The hospital came on board early. I pursued a strategy of growing the trauma program in small steps to improve clinical service and care. I never forced the issue by making the hospital answer the question: "Do you want a trauma center?" I was afraid that if I forced the question before there was a true understanding of the implications of the answer, I could possibly set the program back years. Therefore, accepting progress by growth in small steps turned out to be a winning strategy. One example was to suggest that the hospital supply me with a nurse coordinator by transitioning an existing nursing leadership position in the Emergency Department. The current occupant of that supervisor position had already agreed to be a willing and eager volunteer. Within a relatively short period of time, with multiple presentations to the hospital leadership, the medical staff, and groups such as the Planning Committee of the Hospital Board, that part of the hospital's informal educational program was completed. After completing a financial analysis, the hospital administration became my greatest supporter.

The issue of university support was much more challenging to obtain. One of the highest priorities for the University of Medicine and Dentistry of New Jersey at that time was to have the University Hospital in Newark become financially successful. Having victims of motor vehicle trauma from central New Jersey transported to northern New Jersey's University Hospital seemed like a potential help for that problem. To me, it seemed that having a geographically closer trauma center dedicated to the 2.5 million residents of central New Jersey would result in better care for the acutely injured in that region.

I frequently found myself getting in trouble with the University. The politics were such that the designation process for trauma centers in New Jersey remained in the demonstration phase. It would take statewide political efforts to get the process opened. I always suspected that a front-page article in the statewide newspaper on the efforts to develop a trauma center at Robert Wood Johnson University Hospital was not met with enthusiasm at the headquarters of the University of Medicine and Dentistry of New Jersey in Newark. After we cared for a Rutgers football player and became friendly with the head coach, he offered to connect us to a state legislator. That local politician introduced a bill to open the trauma center designation process. The bill was squashed quickly, and I again had my "hand slapped" by the university. I learned the lesson that there were no shortcuts to getting my superiors on board, and my calling an "end around play" did not help.

My trauma colleague in Newark, Dr. Kenneth Swan, suggested that I be appointed as the next state chair of the American College of Surgeons Committee on Trauma (ACS COT) after his term ended. The ACS COT had both national members and state trauma chair members. When I attended my first national meeting, I learned about the efforts to link rural hospitals to a trauma network. I borrowed the rural concept of trauma regionalization and applied it to suburban central New Jersey. It gave me the idea that my next strategic step should be to create a voluntary trauma network in central New Jersey. Our hospital administration loved the idea. We targeted three nearby hospitals, Somerset Hospital, Perth Amboy General, and Helene Fuld Hospital in Trenton, as potential members of Robert Wood Johnson University Hospital. The premise for joining the Central New Jersey Trauma Network was simple: All the affiliated hospitals could potentially keep the patients they were able to offer quality trauma care and would transfer to RWJUH those that needed care in a Level 1 type trauma center. All hospital members would have to agree to cooperate in the quality case reviews. We submitted a grant to the Robert Wood Johnson Foundation to fund the network's creation and to support an administrative staff. Also included in the funding was money for a heliport for each of the hospitals. We were successful in obtaining the Foundation grant funding for over 1.5 million dollars. In retrospect, I think that more important than the actual funding was the legitimacy conferred by receiving the grant from that national philanthropic agency!

The final piece that directly led to programmatic success was the recruitment of a new CEO for the hospital, who prided himself on his ability to navigate the statewide politics of New Jersey. At my initial meeting with Mr. Harvey Holtzberg, he promised that he could get the state to open the trauma center designation process. He was as good as his word: He worked behind the scenes, did his political magic, and the process was finally opened. The hospital received its Level 1 Trauma Center designation.

The above description of the development of the Trauma Center from de novo idea to fruition took over 9 years. Progress came in fits and starts; tiny progress was followed by setbacks. At times, I was depressed at the slow progress; at other times, I felt euphoria with the possibilities and as we became closer to success. My patience, strained as it was, had paid off mightily.

Lessons Learned on Starting a New Program

1. As I stated above, this was an atypical situation, as most new programs begin with institutional support before the leader starts his assignment of program building. Resources and commitment to the program are usually in place at the inception. As I look back on the experience of building this program, I can identify several lessons: The most important starts with how much can be accomplished through positive interactions with superiors and peers.
2. Lead down by creating a team that focuses primarily on doing the work of improving care. Have ready volunteers who have bought into the vision. Do your best to reinforce the shared successes with shared praise. Improving the care is the best proof of concept.
3. Effectively lead sideways by getting peers on board. Hold discussions that expose the barriers that concern your peers. Address those barriers directly, honestly, and focus on the benefits of cooperation. The key is to create win-win situations.
4. Learning to lead up frequently is the most challenging task. Hospitals and universities have their own priority lists. Play the long game and be persistent as you learn to understand where your program is on the list and formulate a strategy to move it up by convincing leadership of the benefits. Slow and steady progress is fine, but is important to publicly control frustrations. Avoid at all costs burning your own bridges by being labeled a hot-headed jerk.

Reference

1. Hospital and prehospital resources for optimal care of the injured patient. Committee on Trauma of the American College of Surgeons. Bull Am Coll Surg. 1986;71(10):4–23.

Chapter 8
Becoming a Successful Leader of an Established Program

Accepting the position as the new leader of an established program can be very challenging, particularly if the new leader comes from outside the organization. The new leader coming from outside must overcome the "outsider" label. Every institution has its own culture that is woven into the fabric of that institution. There will be an "old guard" that has functioned in a certain manner for years and may not be amenable to change. There may be institutional idiosyncrasies that shaped the introduction of the program. These must be discovered as early as possible. They can easily become unexpected land mines whose detonation will be counterproductive.

Getting promoted from within the institution may have advantages, such as an understanding of the members' personalities and the established culture. On the other hand, the in-house new leader's personal history may also contain unhelpful historical baggage that is forever present, inhibiting success.

I had four opportunities to lead established programs as the "New Guy." The first one was as the new Chief of the Trauma Service at the Kings County Hospital Center in Brooklyn, New York City. The second opportunity was as Chief of Trauma and Surgical Critical Care at the Medical College of Pennsylvania and its hospital system, Allegheny Health Education and Research Foundation (AHERF). The third occurred just about 2 years later when Hahnemann University Hospital joined the AHERF system; I then became the Regional Chief of Trauma for the system and the Chief of Trauma and Surgical Critical Care at both MCP and Hahnemann. The last opportunity came when I was recruited back to Robert Wood Johnson Medical School as Chief of the Division of General Surgery and Robert Wood Johnson University Hospital as the Chief of Surgical Services.

I again had to learn by trial and error, through observation and self-evaluation, what obviously did not work well in my role as the new leader. Over the last 40 years, I have observed new leaders, coming from the outside, take over programs, divisions, and departments. One trend that I witnessed repeatedly was that the new leader came in and utilized the strategy of rapidly "cleaning house," bringing in either old friends or acquaintances as new hires that they trusted, to help rebuild the program. Repeatedly, I saw this strategy fail and lead to the new leader's loss of reputation and ultimate failure. For example, when I was at AHERF in Philadelphia, I saw a newly hired Chair of Orthopedics force out the current, busiest orthopedic specialist at MCP Hospital to bring in his "own loyal people" as one of his first endeavors. He purposefully withdrew and withheld resources from this loyal, busy practitioner whose only crime was that he liked to speak his mind. The new chief assured the hospital administration that he could easily replace the volume. The busy orthopedist eventually left the institution, and the clinical volume was never replaced. The loss of the clinical volume in this and other services eventually resulted in the hospital closure.

The new leader may hold the premise that the old guard is "just terrible" and is not redeemable. This is a common shortcut to create a team with unquestioned loyalty. When the new leader starts with a virtually empty division or department, recruitment of loyal members may be a perfectly acceptable strategy. Under that circumstance, the new leader can and should fill vacant positions as soon as possible. Under most other circumstances, attempts at wholesale replacement of institutionally loyal, competent clinicians and employees create havoc. If the department is populated by expertise or those with successful practices, the "replacement for loyalty" strategy will always fail. The concept that the institution's administrative leadership will accept, without question, even a short-term loss of volume for long-term gain is a recipe for new leader failure. First, large practices with their established referral bases do not come with a guarantee that patients referred will continue to flow after removing their long-time friendly surgeon. The referring physician's reaction is more likely to be one of anger and resulting loss of patient volume that cannot be easily replaced. Hospital administrators do not like losing referrals. It is also a demonstration that the newly recruited leader is a disruptor and not a builder. For the team members, it creates distrust and fear that they are not safe and could be the next to go! I have seen this fail at many of the institutions that I have been associated with, and it never works.

One of the first lessons that I learned as a "new leader" from the outside was that I should proceed slowly. It is better to get to know your new team and new institution's culture before making radical changes. I found that taking on the responsibilities of leading a well-established trauma program at Kings County Hospital Center (The County) in Brooklyn was downright scary. This place had a reputation for being one of the oldest and busiest trauma centers in the country, with a high-profile national reputation for quality care and innovation. I came in with the mandate to essentially "get the trauma docs to play better in the sand box." As a city-run hospital, there were major infrastructure issues that were going to be difficult, if not impossible, for me to improve or fix. Supply chain issues were longstanding and rampant. The physical plant was antiquated and created its own problems. For example, the blood bank was in a different building, and we literally had to send a runner to pick up a batch of units of blood products when needed. Even the act of picking up the blood was complicated and required a knowledgeable currier who arrived at the blood bank with the correct information and requisition slips. It took me months to understand the many work-arounds for transfusions that had developed over the years to enable rapid and effective resuscitations.

I had to be concerned that any changes I might make would have unintended consequences that would slow down the process or even adversely impact other processes that I had not even considered. Ultimately, it could negatively affect patient care. My strategy as the "new guy" was to identify low-hanging fruit that I could easily understand and use to make incremental clinical improvements. I therefore started by establishing my clinical bona fides. During that time, I attempted to demonstrate that I was the real deal; that I was slick in the operating room, knew how to manage injuries, and was willing to learn the Kings County way of managing complicated injuries. I wanted my new colleagues to know that I was open to their input.

In 1989, the trauma surgeons at The County had a different scope of practice than I had in New Brunswick, New Jersey at RWJUH. It was routine for the trauma surgeons at The County to handle more injuries primarily, without help from surgical subspecialists, specifically those in thoracic, vascular, and urologic surgery. At Robert Wood Johnson, I always consulted these subspecialists. I had not operated on injuries in those areas in the 9 years since I was a chief resident at Bellevue. I would need to learn from my new colleagues how to handle those injuries solo. In time, they eventually taught me well.

On my first night on call at The County as the new Chief of the Trauma Service, a patient came in with a trans pelvic gunshot injury with a rectal injury. When taking a trauma night on call, one never knows ahead of time how the patient will present and what the injuries may be. I was fortunate that this patient presented with an injury that I had previously dealt with on numerous occasions. The operation went very well. I remember finishing the operation and, at about 8:00 a.m. the next morning, walking across Clarkson Avenue to Downstate, taking the elevator up to the Department of Surgery offices and seeing my chairman. He congratulated me on how well my first case went and that the residents were impressed! There is a saying: "You only get one chance to make a first impression." I had made the most of mine.

I also found more low-hanging fruit by focusing on creating a Trauma Registry. A Trauma Registry is a list of every patient treated and their demographic data, including mechanism of injury, pre-existing conditions, and outcomes. It is a necessary tool for any quality improvement efforts. To my surprise, a Trauma Registry was not something that existed prior to my tenure. I was creating a great value-added process for the team to see. I also created a special separate registry to track our care of patients with extremity injuries related to firearms. This allowed us, as a group to do a prospective study [1]. My initial strategies were therefore deliberately focused on improving patient care by creating registries and contributing to our research efforts. It was very gratifying that these efforts yielded some early successes.

I do have to admit that it was not totally a smooth sail down a calm river. I had my missteps as well. Just prior to taking the position of Trauma Chief at The County, I had published a simplified surgical technique for operative repair of the injured spleen. It was well-received nationally. At that time, the County was one of the pioneers in developing strategies for the non-operative management of isolated splenic trauma, employing selective proximal splenic artery embolization. These efforts were led by an innovative interventional radiologist who was revolutionizing the non-operative management of many injuries. I was unfamiliar with The County's unwritten protocol for splenic management. This radiologist became personally offended when I did a splenic repair operatively. He did let me know of his upset, and I subsequently adopted the The County way of managing splenic injuries with his involvement. He later admitted that he was so upset with me after I operatively repaired an injured spleen, that he interfered, as a member of the Appointment and Promotions Committee at Downstate, with my academic appointment. For all the 3 years that I spent at The County and Downstate, my faculty appointment never was approved, and I remained Professor of Surgery (Visiting).

My experiences at AHERF in 1993 as the new leader of the Trauma and Surgical Critical Care Service at the Medical College of Pennsylvania Hospital (MCPH) followed a similar pattern. I started slowly, tried to learn the culture, and began with what I perceived would be potential easy wins. My initial responsibility was at one hospital, the Medical College of Pennsylvania Hospital. Shortly thereafter, the system absorbed Hahnemann University Hospital, which had its own Level 1 Trauma Center. My assignment, as the system and the medical school chief, became to meld the two Trauma Level 1 Centers into one. Each Trauma Center had a distinct and very different culture.

At MCPH, the strength was the front door and the Emergency Department. MCPH was the birthplace of the discipline of Emergency Medicine. The specialty was carved out from the turf of other departments. Their leader, Dr. David Wagner, was in fact a board-certified pediatric surgeon. My initial impression of him was that he was a kind man and above all else a gentleman. The Emergency Department had wonderful clinicians with very strong personalities. They were involved in every phase of the resuscitation of the acutely injured. The Emergency Department physicians had been very supportive of my predecessor in the establishment of the Level 1 Trauma Center. They dominated all issues related to trauma resuscitations.

As I assessed the functioning of the Trauma Center, I concluded that we needed more involvement of experts from other departments. Very early on, I had to deal with an issue that involved balancing the need to train Emergency Medicine residents in airway management and the needs of the trauma patient with a difficult airway, in extremis, who would benefit from having the most experienced individual dealing with the airway. In brief, I thought we should have more involvement of the Anesthesia Service in difficult airway management. There was a red line drawn with tape on the floor of the resuscitation area. Anesthesia personnel could not cross that red line, as they had no assigned role! After considerable pushback from the ED docs, I negotiated a solution that had the anesthesiologists teach the Emergency Medicine residents airway management.

The culture at Hahnemann University Hospital was quite different from that at MCPH. Hahnemann Hospital has a long history of organized trauma care. Under their chair, Dr. Charles Wolfreth, they were one of the first designated Level 1

Trauma Centers in the Commonwealth of Pennsylvania. At the time Hahnemann joined the Allegheny System, Dr. Wolfreth had long since left, and the trauma program was in disarray. Their last trauma chief had recently moved on, and the program barely had enough general surgeons volunteering to take trauma calls. There were only a few dedicated trauma and critical care surgeons involved. The administrative leadership, infrastructure, and support for the program via the nursing service and educational program remained very strong.

The general surgical residencies of MCPH and Hahnemann up to then were independent and had been combined by the merger. It appeared to me, as the new leader, that the low-hanging fruit was to build the same new trauma infrastructure for both programs. This was crucial because now general surgery residents were spending time in both institutions. In fact, a real patient safety issue had been created by the previous terminology used for triage. The same words used to describe levels of resuscitation (triage criteria) had a different meaning at MCPH and Hahnemann Hospital. We instituted standardized nomenclature for classifying resuscitation categories and clinical protocols at both institutions to avoid confusion [2]. The exercises to create common infrastructure and protocols involved the medical and nursing staff at both institutions and were the first steps to establishing the new culture. I created the positions of Associate Chief of Trauma and Surgical Critical Care at each hospital, which reported directly to me. The site leader at MCPH was appointed from the existing faculty, and we recruited a site leader for Hahnemann quickly. We had combined conferences that were well attended. I also decided to take trauma calls at both sites and lead rounds in both intensive care units. All of the above turned out to be effective first steps.

At both sites, the trauma surgeons and residents functioned quite well and behaved as members of the same integrated team. The other staff with a long history of being aligned with their respective institutions were less flexible. I appreciated the institutional pride at Hahnemann as being one of the first trauma centers in the city and the commonwealth, as well as the fact that they had their own helicopter and trauma fellowship. The Hahnemann group had the feeling that they were the victims of a hostile takeover by a "lesser" program.

The Allegheny leadership wanted a regional trauma program but unfortunately did not create a common budget. Each of the trauma center's finances remained integrated into their respective hospital's budget processes. When I studied the individual profit and loss analysis for each of the programs, I noted that MCPH's Level 1 Trauma Center lost money while Hahnemann's was profitable. The local catchment area for trauma patients was similar in terms of payor status, but the helicopter brought in some better-remunerating patients from the suburbs to Hahnemann. A deeper dive into the finances revealed other more important reasons for the disparity in profitability. It came down to the allocation of expenses. MCPH pooled all the surgical service's expenses and allocated an average dollar expense per surgical patient. This resulted in an artificially decreased expense per patient for the cardiac surgery program while arbitrarily increasing the expense for the trauma patients. In addition, the expense of any 24/7 hospital resource required for trauma center designation was allocated directly to the trauma center budget line, even if utilized by other services. The blood bank was an example of this. Any operational upgraded services, such as the Blood Bank or Operating Room staff, were a line item for the Trauma Center at MCPH. For Hahnemann, it was not applied just to the Trauma Center budget line, as it was recognized that other services such as the cardiac and transplant services benefited from the 24/7 coverage in the blood bank and operating room.

I placed the barrier of the financial disparity and lack of a combined budget on my long-range list of "to do issues" that was going to take a more long-term solution. It did create problems with the distribution of helicopter patients. Bringing patients transported to MCPH by helicopter always came with massive pushback. Unfortunately, AHERF underwent bankruptcy, and I never had the opportunity to deal with long-term issues and fully integrate the finances of the two programs.

Lessons Learned to be a Successful New Leader of an Established Program

1. First and foremost, demonstrate emotional intelligence and character. For clinicians, it will be important to remember that "eyes" are always on you.
2. Get your "hands dirty" with clinical activity. It is the only way to learn about the culture, strengths, and weaknesses of your new home. Demonstration of expertise leads to immediate credibility. You need to establish yourself as the champion of quality care and to personally be able to deliver that quality. Avoid being arrogant and be ready to learn from the expertise that is already present. Try to establish yourself as a transformational leader. Seek advice from the old guard in public forums, in open meetings, while you attempt to build consensus.
3. Assess the culture of the new institution before making any drastic or even dramatic changes. Try to understand how your proposed major changes might have predictable and unpredictable outcomes. Minimize the opportunity for unanticipated outcomes that your changes may bring. This can only be accomplished by fully understanding the system you're inheriting. Listen to your team and glean from them what they think are important changes and expected outcomes. That kind of behavior will win you the respect of the team and allow you to develop the concept of shared responsibility. It will also prevent you from making some obvious errors.
4. At the same time, it is appropriate to point out the opportunities for improvement and get the entire team involved in the process of improvement. This demonstrates your commitment to quality and the will to improve outcomes. What if the "old guard" is resistant to change? First, go for the low-hanging fruit. After demonstrating clinical expertise, start the process of change by taking on low-risk, high-reward areas like educational programs and improving simple protocols. Only after achieving some major victories and demonstrating that your goal is to be inclusive should you tackle the more controversial and difficult issues.

5. How do you deal with uncooperative team members? That team member may also be an individual who was the in-house candidate for the job that you have just started. They may want to see you fail! This will take excellence in leading down and sidewise to its limits. The strategy for success is to play the long game. Always stake out the high ground by focusing on improving quality. It is important to treat all team members equally and with respect, whether they agree or not or whether they cooperate fully or not. This approach can be very challenging and will take some time to bear fruit, but it can work and lead to sustained success.

References

1. Trooskin SZ, Sclafani S, Winfield J, Duncan AO, Scalea T, Vieux E, Atweh N, Gertler J. The management of vascular injuries of the extremity associated with civilian firearms. Surg Gynecol Obstet. 1993 Apr;176(4):350–4.
2. Trooskin SZ, Faucher MB, Santora TA, Talucci RC. Consolidation of trauma programs in the era of large health care delivery networks. J Trauma. 1999 Mar;46(3):488–93.

Chapter 9
Medical School Leadership: Department of Surgery Division Chief or Chair

Being a leader of a division or department chair offers additional and somewhat unique challenges. There is a need for expertise in diverse and seemingly unrelated responsibilities. Leadership is required for the clinical enterprise, research efforts, the educational programs, and the academic and personal advancement of the faculty. Leading the clinical enterprise by itself is a difficult and complex job. The Chief or Chair will have to lead the research efforts of the division or department. Some leaders will have their own successful lab with grants or a successful clinical research enterprise. At the very least, the leader must create an environment fostering the research success of the students, residents, and faculty. The educational mission spans the arc of program requirements for medical students, surgical residents, and fellows as well as the faculty. He or she is also responsible for recruitment of new faculty and retention of valuable faculty. Finally, the leader is responsible for faculty development. Some faculty will have career aspirations in the different arenas of clinical activity, bench research, and some as master educators. The faculty will need mentoring at frequent intervals to achieve their potential for maximum growth. It is a daunting task to do this leadership job well.

Do today's leaders have to be "triple threats"? Do they have to be stars in all the arenas of clinical care, research, and administration? Historically, the answer was yes. In today's environment, with NIH money subject to extreme competition, it is difficult to maintain a busy practice, provide administrative leadership, and compete with full-time researchers in other disciplines. There are very few successful researchers with busy clinical practices. Therefore, there are many pathways to becoming a chair of a department of surgery. It is no longer necessary to be a triple threat in all the above areas. Some chairs earn their position via excellence in program development and/or are national clinical innovators.

No matter how one obtained the position, the key to having a successful chairmanship is to become a successful administrator and leader. Demonstration of character and emotional intelligence are the prime ingredients for success. One can become a surgical chair because of clinical expertise and perform operations that

S. Z. Trooskin, *An Introduction to Medical Leadership for Surgeons*, https://doi.org/10.1007/978-3-031-44264-3_9

few can do, but without the ability to interact successfully with superiors, department members, residents, and students, the individual in the administrative role will fail. It is more important than the attributes that secure the position.

I was blessed by having been exposed to a variety of Chair role models with different styles of leadership. The first chairman I observed, as a fourth-year medical student, was Dr. Henry T. Bahnson, a noted cardiac surgeon at the University of Pittsburgh School of Medicine. In 1974, I did not realize at the time he was demonstrating emotional intelligence in all his interactions. What I witnessed was a calm, dignified, knowledgeable surgeon who always behaved like a gentleman. He was a great teacher in the operating room. He had the ability to direct his teaching efforts to the appropriate level for each member of the team. In that era, at the University of Pittsburgh, the patient was placed on cardiopulmonary bypass via the femoral artery and vein. Dr. Bahnson personally instructed the cardiac surgery fellow in the most critical cardiac portion of the operation with a controlled calmness. He taught the junior resident how to repair the femoral arteriotomy, while the cardiothoracic fellow closed the sternum. He saw me struggling when I was tying knots while closing the skin. He called me over after one operation, and we sat in the corner while he taught me some tricks for knot tying. It is no wonder that he became one of my early role models for remaining calm, gentlemanly, and personally relating to the individual team members. I had scrubbed with several surgeons on the faculty who seemed to be very self-absorbed. I could not see aspiring to be like them, but Dr. Bahnson, well, he was different. The biggest lesson I learned from him was to treat team members as individuals, try to understand what they need, and supply it.

The Chair during my surgical residency was Dr. Frank Spencer, who was also a cardiac surgeon. He demanded excellence from himself and everyone around him with an almost monomaniacal passion. Patients at NYU and Bellevue were "not allowed to die." If they died, their surgeon had better know whether it was the technique or the concept that was wrong. The surgeon had to learn what the plan would be for the next time so that the result would be different. Our M&M Conferences on Thursday afternoon were legendary. The room was packed with students, residents, and faculty. Attendance was not taken, but it was understood that unless you were actively involved in saving a life, you had better be there. The chief resident stood in the front of the room just opposite "The Boss" and presented the case. It was not a "kind and gentle" learning experience. On the other hand, it was the most productive hour of learning each week. Sometimes Dr. Spencer would present one of his own cases and analyze it critically. He thus demonstrated that he was not immune to errors and that he also relentlessly ruminated about what he could do better for the next patient. If the chief resident had not demonstrated what he learned from the complication, "The Boss" did not hide his anger, and the spectacle of public embarrassment would begin. The best way to avoid public humiliation at those M&M Conferences was to come prepared and own the responsibility for the complication and to have figure out the best approach to avoid the same unwanted result next time.

"The Boss" was a man to be revered and feared at the same time. If a chief resident presented a case and did not analyze it thoroughly, public humiliation soon followed. It could get very ugly and downright embarrassing. There were some specific errors that could predictably bring out that type of response from "The Boss." He would not tolerate basic care delivered inferiorly. Nothing would bring out his anger more than losing control of a patient's airway. He would ask the chief resident presenting, "Did you like this man?" and worse if he got on a roll. Thankfully, those occasions were rare. Most frequently, he would come up with excellent teaching points.

I remember a particular case from when I was the chief resident of the Trauma Service. A patient came in with stab wounds in the right upper quadrant and left lower quadrant. He was in extremis, and we took him immediately to the operating room. I performed a laparotomy incision and could not evacuate the blood fast enough to see anything, as he was exsanguinating from injuries to the bifurcation of the hepatic and portal veins and the hepatic artery. I opened his left chest and cross-clamped his aorta. I, to this day, remember the two teaching points. One was that I should have compressed the abdominal aorta at the level of the diaphragm with my hand or a bulky retractor. It would have been more efficient than opening the chest. That teaching point saved lives over the course of my career as a trauma surgeon. The second teaching point was that I should have called the attending who was an expert in the management of liver trauma instead of, or in addition to, the attending surgeon on call. As M&M Conferences go, I handled myself well and was not embarrassed. But right after the conference, as Dr. Spencer and I were walking to his office to have our weekly chiefs meeting, he said to me, "Stan, I can't believe that you let that man bleed to death." I interpreted that as a devastating comment, that I had disappointed "The Boss" by having the patient die. It took me a while to get over those words.

A few years later, when I was a junior attending on call at RWJUH, a patient came in with devastating liver injury that I managed without errors, and the patient did great. As I thought about the case and analyzed it, my mind flashed back to that chief resident presentation I made at the M&M Conference, and I compared the two cases. By then, I had gained more experience, and it dawned on me that my case as a chief resident was unsalvageable, that the patient had lethal injuries that were not survivable. "The Boss" was teasing me by telling me, in a way he thought I would understand, that the patient could not be saved. I do not think he appreciated my still clinical naiveté, that my respect for him was so deep, that I interpreted his comments literally and was crushed by them. I learned that the words of the leader could be misinterpreted and could have untoward effects.

I have had the opportunity to attend M&M Conferences over the entirety of my career and to lead them for over 25 years. Never have I seen an entire department so dedicated to improving clinical outcomes as I had witnessed as a resident at NYU. The motivation for this was the leadership of Dr. Spencer and his personal quest for excellence and perfection. How much was also related to the fear of public humiliation or fear of losing the respect of "The Boss"? I have no doubt that much of the department took great pride in their outcomes. They truly believed they were the best surgeons working in the best department in the country. I also appreciated that fear was also a defining motivation for several of the surgical residents and faculty as well. The culture of excellence started at the top.

The environment and the style of the M&M Conferences at NYU had their origins at Johns Hopkins in the late nineteenth century and the chairman William Stewart Halsted. I could find no direct evidence of public humiliation being used as a motivator, but it could have been present at that institution as well. Dr. Bahnson, who also trained there and was a member of the surgical faculty at Hopkins, did not bring that with him to the University of Pittsburgh. Dr. Bahnson recruited another former Hopkins surgeon and leader, Dr. Mark Ravitch, to his department in Pittsburgh, after Dr. Ravitch had alienated the faculties at Mount Sinai and the University of Chicago. I attended a resident conference where Dr. Ravitch reviewed the week's Operating Room schedules and called on the residents who scrubbed on those cases. He grilled them on indications, pathophysiology, and surgical technique. It was not a kind and gentle atmosphere. The good aspect of this conference was that it was done behind closed doors, with no departmental audience. Only Dr. Ravitch, the residents, and the medical students were present. It was one of the ways that the department engrained responsibility for the privilege of caring for patients.

When I started to lead my department's quality efforts and M&M Conferences, I wanted to create a more collegial culture of excellence and continuous improvement. In the years after I left my surgical training at NYU and that generation of surgical leaders retired, the tactic of using intimidation as a motivator were also retired. That was a good change.

My initial efforts at leading M&M and starting the process of culture change involved my attempting to incorporate some of the techniques that had worked for me before. First, I tried to be the best role model that I could be. I made sure that my complications were presented, I owned up to my failures, and I clearly delineated what I would do differently. I met with the surgical residents consistently for breakfast for years. Early on in my career, I met with them every weekday. I would have them run the list of patients and present case summaries. I tried to ask probing questions and give feedback. I also tried to keep track of the complications and mortalities by having the residents keep the M&M list and asked them to add cases to the list when appropriate.

The Department of Surgery at Cedars-Sinai Medical Center had developed a program that they labelled The M&M Matrix [1]. It was a method to link their M&M and other resident educational conferences to the surgical literature and their preparation efforts for the American Board of Surgery Qualifying Examination. I shamelessly borrowed from this program. During my years as the general surgery residency program director, I assigned a chief resident to keep the matrix list and the schedule of presentations. This chief resident also circulated a de-identified summary of the teaching points to the department. I never managed to directly link the educational topics from the M&M Conference to the entire resident education curriculum.

I made further adjustments to the M&M Conference to use a type of "intimidation" that did not involve public humiliation. I noticed at times during the conference that the attending surgeons were very defensive and argued the facts of the case with the residents. To combat this, I had the residents submit to me copies of the salient parts of the medical record far in advance of the conference so I could become knowledgeable about the case. The intimidation came into play, as everyone present knew, that I had reviewed the chart. It was then much more difficult to argue the facts with the residents during the conference. I never did achieve the near-perfect attendance by residents and attending surgeons at the M&M Conference that I had witnessed at NYU. To make sure that at least the provider participants consistently attended, I had the residents sign an attestation form that they had personally notified the involved attending of the up-and-coming presentation. In the final years, I began to review the presentation by the residents' pre-conference, one on one, either via phone or in person in my office and tried to draw out their opinions of what was done wrong and what they would do differently. The M&M Conference was a very labor-intense endeavor for me. There were times I longed for the good old days of the authoritative, dogmatic, and scary academic leader.

Recruitment Strategies for Division Chiefs and Chairs

Over my long career, I have had the experience of working in different sized departments, small, medium, and large. With those experiences, I have come to several conclusions. In a department or division, faculty should be equally divided at junior, intermediate, and senior career levels. This construction will provide many advantages for the department. Senior members supply role models for the entire group and provide experienced clinical, leadership, or research expertise. In academic surgery, a leader must accept that faculty will move on, therefore having depth in subspecialties is an important goal. Depth at the various levels will allow the clinical programs to go on when faculty leave. It also implies, for the faculty, that you can grow and advance locally.

Recruiting faculty can be quite challenging. To be perfectly honest, I believe that I was only marginally effective at recruiting new faculty and not particularly good at consistently selecting the right individuals from outside the institution. I did better, for the most part, in evaluating whether my own surgical residents would make excellent additions to the faculty. Having worked with them day in and day out, I had more than a reasonable understanding of their strengths and weaknesses.

When recruiting from the outside, I had difficulty in evaluating, during the recruitment process, the strengths and more importantly the weaknesses of a given candidate. One exception was a gentleman, an interventional gastroenterologist, who was a "throw in" as his wife, a radiation oncologist, was being recruited, and her husband was invited to meet with me in my role as Chief of the Division of General Surgery at Robert Wood Johnson School of Medicine. The first thing that I noticed was that he had a skill set that was not available currently in our gastroenterology group. Secondly, we bonded immediately as I could see that he had a terrific work ethic, calm demeanor, and was a gentleman. It turned out to be a great hire. We collaborated closely during his entire tenure with us, our patients received great care, and it was a pleasure to work with him. My initial impression of him was correct in all aspects.

Unfortunately, I also recruited individuals with great reputations and a decent track record of success who turned out to be a poor fit with the environment and culture. Some recruits could not deal with the frustrations of a slower-moving bureaucracy than they had experienced in their previous institutions. Others had issues with interpersonal skills that were not reflected in their glowing recommendations. I swung and missed with an early trauma recruit. His recommendations were stellar, and he was a decent clinician. Unfortunately, he had a very short temper and a propensity to frequently pepper his conversations with four letter expletives at the worst times.

Having had experiences of missing key traits in recruits more than once, I would suggest that the surgical leader put together an ad hoc recruitment committee. Trusted department or division members and some from outside the department/division should be invited to participate in the process. I would not just rely on the interviewer completing a form but having a meeting or meetings with the committee. The chief would be well served by empowering that group to do a thorough dive into the candidate's background and previous experiences. There will be the added benefits of involving more people in the process and enhancing ownership in the department's decision-making.

The surgical leader should keep in mind that recruitment of mid-level or senior faculty may have a ripple effect on other members of the faculty division members. The recruitment of highly qualified individuals will require the devotion of considerable resources for salary and program development that may upset the current balance. The established faculty may feel underappreciated. The fallout will have to be dealt with and retention strategies initiated.

Faculty Retention Strategies for Division Chiefs and Surgical Chairs

Not counting my own surgical residency, I have closely observed six individuals who held the position of Chair of the department; this is in addition to the two interim chairs that I observed up close and my own personal experience as an interim chair. The key to retaining valued faculty is to make sure the faculty feel that they are appreciated. There are two ways to accomplish this. The first is to ensure that the faculty hear from the chief, on a frequent basis, that they are appreciated. The second is to be able to provide the appropriate remuneration or salary. In the present environment, the former resides within the capacity of the chief or chair. The latter is much more complicated, as it requires the chair to come up with more resources that he/she may have to secure from their immediate superior, the department chair for division chief, and the dean of the medical school for the chair.

Expressing appreciation and confirming job security is not expensive but does require the investment of the leader's time and attentiveness. The time spent needs to be one on one. The two of my chairs that I thought did this the most effectively were Dr. Bernie Jaffe and Dr. Stephen Lowry. Dr. Jaffe, my Chair at Downstate, spent a lot of time with his faculty. He knew their personal stories, their wives, and their families in a depth that I had never experienced before I met him. He and his wife, Marlene, developed a close relationship with my wife and family. I was invited to his home and he came to mine. I think the man never slept, as I would hear from him at odd hours of the night. He sought out my opinion on departmental matters and made me feel that my input was important to the decision-making process. He had an outsized, gregarious personality and used it to get departmental information that he valued.

Dr. Lowry, my Chair at Robert Wood Johnson Medical School, was just terrific to spend time with one on one. He was not exceptionally outgoing, but he was not shy either. There was little informal socializing outside of work, but he had the exceptional characteristic of projecting his honest interest in his faculty. It was palpable. He had the ability to listen attentively and to make each of the faculty feel that he appreciated their contribution. I used to leave our meetings feeling valued by my chair as one of the most important members of the department. I was not alone in feeling that way.

Dealing with salary increase requests was one of the most difficult issues that I had to deal with as both a Division Chief and Interim Chair. Most times, the needed resources were not under my direct access but were controlled by my supervisors. Additionally, raising salaries under ordinary circumstances can take time. To deal with this successfully, the Chair must keep the faculty member informed of the process and the status of the request. The faculty member must believe that the Chair or Chief is acting as an advocate and really cares. Advocacy must be presented in a language that demonstrates value. The Chair must also use logic in making the case with the Dean or Hospital CEO. Deans understand productivity in terms of clinical income, RVUs, program development, and grant funding. Hospital administrators understand the contribution to margin and hate to lose those faculty that contribute to the bottom line. Chairs can be faced with valued faculty that have an offer in hand. If that is the case, the Chair must convey the sense of urgency to the Dean and hospital leaders. It is sometimes helpful to have those leaders meet directly with the faculty members. Some Chairs are overly sensitive for faculty members to meet with those individuals. My feeling is that, as the leader, I should set up the appointment and set the stage for the Dean and/or the hospital president. That way, it was not an "end around maneuver," and I could continue to be in control of the process. Close follow-up after those meetings is important as well. The process of putting together a counteroffer must get into gear very quickly as time is usually of the essence. The faculty member will be under a time limit to respond to the offer and coming back with the counteroffer will demonstrate institutional commitment.

The Role of the Chair and Division Chiefs in Mentoring Students

One of the most important aspects of academic leadership is mentoring. This function, to my view, is the easiest to scrimp on in terms of spending time and effort but should be one of the highest priorities for the chair or division chief. It is the best investment for the long-term health of the department or the division. It involves putting aside time to meet with medical students, surgical residents, and all levels of the faculty.

The Chair should be inspiring medical students to choose a career in surgery and to help them reach their goals. As a medical student, I was inspired by the gentlemanly Dr. Bahnson. I observed two Chairs do this exceptionally well: Dr. Frank Spencer and Dr. Bernard Jaffe. Dr. Jaffe would meet with each new group of students on the first morning of their surgery clerkship and give introductory remarks in addition to at least one lecture in his area of expertise. He made himself imminently approachable. He had an open-door policy for students and invited them to work on research projects. Those students interested in surgery would get his attention and help with a personal letter of recommendation.

Dr. Spencer utilized his photographic memory at the beginning of his monthly lectures to go down the list of students on that surgical clerkship so that he could link a name to a face. No notes were necessary for him to accomplish this. It was the job of the Administrative Chief Resident to escort "The Boss" from his office to the lecture room in Bellevue. I do not recall specifically how he advised medical students who showed an interest in surgery. I do recall that he knew the NYU medical students who stayed for their surgical residency very well.

I have seen different methods for authoring Chair's letters for residency recommendation. Some department chairs will author their own letter or assign a faculty member to write a composite letter that the Chair either signs or co-signs with the real author. There is no doubt that the students know the methodology. The fact is that the more the Chair is involved in the letter, the more impressed the medical students will be. At a minimum, the Chair needs to meet with all those medical students applying for surgical residency and interact personally at least one time. The key to satisfactorily mentoring medical students then is to be an excellent role model and be available to interact with them personally.

The Role of the Chairs and Division Chiefs in Mentoring Residents

The Chair does have the responsibility to mentor residents. Although there is always a premium on the time of the leader, the time spent with trainees is time well spent. Different Chairs have employed different styles to interact with residents. If the Chair is a general surgeon, the Chair can make professor rounds at scheduled intervals. Likewise, the Chair, if in a different clinical discipline, can set up meetings at predictable intervals. I remember a story that Dr. John Landor, my first Chief of General Surgery at Rutgers Medical School, once told me about his Chair, Dr. Lester Dragsted. Dr. Dragsted would have afternoon tea once a week with the residents. I suspect that was done very frequently 70 years ago. In our current age, breakfast before the operating room schedule begins or dinner off-site would probably be more effective.

The Chair and the Division Chiefs must create an environment for academic curiosity and encourage both clinical and laboratory research. The leaders should financially support resident travel to present their research projects and reinforce the success. A Resident Research Day event is a terrific venue for the residents to present their laboratory and clinical projects. It was established for the Department of Surgery at Rutgers Robert Wood Johnson Medical School by Dr. Nell Maloney Patel, the General Surgery Residency Program Director, and Dr. Leonard Lee, the current Chair of Surgery. In that program, all general surgery residents are required to complete at least one project per academic year. It can be a case study, clinical review, prospective or retrospective clinical study, or a basic laboratory research project. The clinical and laboratory categories are set up as a competition; the top three papers in each category are presented orally to the department, and the remaining are presented as posters. Judges are assigned to rank the papers. It is also open to all divisions in the department. Events like this demonstrate the department's and in particular the Chair's commitment to academic excellence.

Facilitating the residents' involvement with quality improvement is also an opportunity for mentoring. Starting to involve residents in quality improvement projects early on in their training will prepare them for future involvement throughout their careers. The ACGME has been monitoring resident involvement in hospital governance and quality programs via the CLER Program [2]. As Surgical Service Chief, a few years ago, I created a continuous hospital based quality program for the General Surgical Residency that was integrated into the Peri-operative Surgical Services Quality Program. Each of the six surgical chief residents was placed in charge of a quality team that consisted of a resident representative for each categorical clinical year. The teams were designed to have continuity: When the present chief resident graduates, the former PGY-4, now the new chief resident, takes over leadership of the projects. In the beginning, each team was tasked to identify a few projects that they wanted to work on to improve clinical outcomes. Meetings were held with all the residents to discuss the proposed projects and to ensure that they were being guided by faculty to narrow the scope and define deliverables.

The initial meetings were fascinating. First, the residents identified important and meaningful issues for improvement. Second, they initially voiced a lot of frustration at the slowness of progress. We dealt with this by reminding them that these were long-term important projects and underscored the incremental progress that was being made. In the first few years, this program became a huge success. The residents' quality work led to tangible improvements in clinical care at Robert Wood Johnson University Hospital. The general surgery residents initiated and then achieved the transition in the hospital, from utilizing resident pagers to cell phones;

they also successfully developed and initiated a half dozen clinical protocols and pathways for outcome improvement. They learned that quality improvement efforts can succeed with their active involvement. They also had the opportunity to present some of their successes at a national meeting.

The Role of Chairs and Division Chiefs in Mentoring Faculty

I was quite fortunate as a junior faculty member at Rutgers Medical School in 1980 to have had tremendous mentorship. They were Dr. John Landor, the then Chief of General Surgery, who recruited me, and his successor, Dr. Ralph Greco. Both gentlemen have since passed and are greatly missed by the generations of students and residents that they trained. Although not national power brokers, they were outstanding mentors. From the moment that I started at Rutgers Medical School after completing general surgery training, they clearly articulated what I needed to accomplish to have a successful academic career. Dr. Landor was the quintessential academic surgeon and was also the mentor to Dr. Greco. Dr. Landor's career was built on the classic design of developing a successful laboratory research portfolio, clinical expertise, and successive administrative responsibilities.

Dr. Landor, under the tutelage of his Chair, Dr. Lester Dragsted, became a nationally respected expert in gastric acid secretion physiology and the etiology of peptic ulcer disease. He was an excellent clinician who taught me many subtle clinical "pearls" and surgical techniques, including how to consistently identify the recurrent laryngeal nerve. He did have one Achilles heel: He could not tolerate "fools." As Chief of the Division of General Surgery and Residency Program Director at the then Rutgers Medical School, he attempted to coordinate the residents' clinic schedule with Operating Room block time assignments. This was in the early days of the conversion of the hospital from a community hospital to a primary medical school teaching hospital. The Operating Room Committee pushed back on his efforts. In anger, he resigned from his position as Chief of General Surgery in the weeks just before I was to begin my academic career. He remained on the faculty for 4 years and mentored me in my research projects and clinical efforts. He eventually left to work in a federally funded clinic and hospital serving the indigenous population in New Mexico. He later became Chief of Surgery at the Brooklyn Veterans Hospital, which was part of the Department of Surgery at Downstate. He was serving in that role when I was recruited to the same department in 1989. He continued to mentor me for most of the first half of my career. Interestingly, he did not have the patience for long-term administrative responsibilities and stepped down from that Veterans Hospital position as well.

Dr. Ralph Greco mentored me day-to-day and helped me to build my academic career. When my independent research endeavors stalled, he took me into his lab. My work in his lab resulted in my first Surgical Forum presentation. Not only did he edit the initial draft of my abstract, but he also took me to a large lecture hall to hear a dry run of my presentation. He critiqued my speaking style and counted the number of times I spoke haltingly and said "a." That lesson and others in public speaking served me so very well throughout my career. After the presentation in Atlanta, he took me out to dinner, and we celebrated. It was a model of mentoring that I adopted for my career.

Dr. Greco coached me and monitored my progress in reaching the criteria for promotion up the academic ladder to Associate and then Professor of Surgery. I felt that I was supported in all the basic aspects of my career. When I reached the appropriate number of presentations, publications, and secured a grant to create a trauma network, my application to the Appointment and Promotion Committee as Associate Professor with tenure was approved. These many conversations with my division chiefs that led to my success were specific and my progress was monitored closely. This mentoring resulted in my promotion to Associate Professor with tenure 5 years after first joining the faculty.

I was introduced to the importance of progressing through national surgical organizations. I was given the goals of gaining membership in the Association of Academic Surgery (AAS), the Society of University Surgeons (SUS), and finally into the very competitive American Surgical Association (ASA). From the beginning of my academic career, I knew that one of my ultimate goals was to apply for and to be elected to membership in the ASA, the oldest and most prestigious of all the surgical organizations. Dr. Bernie Jaffe did the same for valued members of his department at Downstate. Unfortunately, since leaving Downstate, I have not seen this type of focused mentoring and detailed coaching that benefits the individual faculty member, the department, and its divisions. More recently, I have seen division chiefs stress the importance of focusing solely on presentations and advancement in subspecialty organizations (e.g., surgical oncology, trauma, or vascular national organizations) as opposed to having their mentees achieve success and advancement in the most prestigious, general national organizations. It is beneficial to the department's national reputation to have members enter the SUS and the ASA.

Faculty need to be mentored in their understanding of a concept that I have labeled as the "currency" for judging success in today's world. I have come to understand that the "currency" for success comes in three modalities. The first is research success in terms of obtaining grant funding. The second is "patient power" or control over a large referral-based practice. The third is expertise in administrative excellence in program building. These types of currency lead to power and influence within the medical school or hospital system. Success in any of these venues can help to create security for the individual faculty or medical staff member. Mentoring young faculty in these very different potential pathways can be very helpful for faculty to plan for their ultimate success.

Lessons Learned for Successful Interactions as a Division Chief/Department Chair

1. The key to becoming successful as a Chief or Chair is to be an effective role model and appropriately direct efforts to the various constituents within the division/department.
2. It is very important to have a plan that focuses on faculty development which includes recruitment, retention, and mentoring.
3. The transformative leader will create a committee system to guide the recruitment process with effective input.
4. Effective retention and mentoring strategies involve interacting personally with the students, residents, and faculty on a consistent basis.
5. In addition to being an effective role model and daily demonstrating character, Chairs and Division Chiefs as leaders need to spell out the criteria for achieving success. They need to monitor progress and be able to help with mid-course corrections.
6. The "old school approach" of spending time with Chair/Division Chief meetings is of paramount importance. The Chair must be that transformative medical leader who both listens to and guides his team members and supports their future ambitions.

References

1. Gordon LA. Can cedars-Sinai's "M+M matrix" save surgical education? Bull Am Coll Surg. 2004 Jun;89(6):16–20.
2. Clinical Learning Environment Review (CLER) (www.acgme.org).

Chapter 10
Branching Out into Hospital Leadership: Elected Positions

The members of hospital medical staff vote on a slate of candidates for their leadership positions of Secretary/Treasurer, Vice President (or President-Elect), and President. When serving as Medical Staff President, it is important to remember this fact. Your major constituency is to represent the medical staff in its interaction with hospital administration to deliver optimal care to the patients. It means that your loyalty primarily belongs to the medical staff when involved in efforts to improve patient care. That said, the medical staff president must have an excellent working relationship with the hospital administration and the clinical department leaders, the Chiefs and Chairs, to carry out this mission effectively. The most effective medical staff presidents that I have witnessed had previously earned and continued to earn the respect of the hospital service leaders while also serving the best interests of the entire medical staff.

I served as Medical Staff President at the Medical College of Pennsylvania Hospital for a term and a half (the previous president holding the position when I was President-Elect was ill, and I had to step into the role of president early). I have also served on the Medical Executive Committee at two university hospitals for over 26 years and have observed many presidents in addition to my own experiences. The most successful medical staff presidents have put doing what was best for the patients as their number one responsibility. They managed the sometimes complicated politics by following that guiding principle.

The potential political issues between hospital administration and medical staff leadership can be protean and challenging. During my first term, I was asked by the CEO of the hospital to deliver a vote at the Medical Executive Committee, which was in the hospital's best interest but was somewhat controversial. Early in my tenure, I was asked to promote it and fast-track its acceptance at the next Med Exec meeting. I attempted to do this, but it was voted down. When I analyzed "my failure," I thought I was reckless in trying to fast-track a controversial issue. In retrospect, I should have fostered a comprehensive discussion. I had potentially placed my credibility with the medical staff leadership at risk. A more appropriate response

S. Z. Trooskin, *An Introduction to Medical Leadership for Surgeons*, https://doi.org/10.1007/978-3-031-44264-3_10

would have been for me to have pushed back on the CEO's request and reminded her that there are no shortcuts to building consensus.

Leading groups of physicians and medical staff have been likened to "herding cats." An excellent medical staff president needs to become an excellent "cat herder." A successful cat herder needs to understand his/her herd and the multiple factions within the herd while accepting a few basic concepts. The first concept is that the medical staff is multidisciplinary; they are not all surgeons or internal medicine docs but represent every medical subspecialty. Each subspecialty will have its own set of priorities. The second is that the medical staff most likely is divided into factions based on how they are remunerated. These generally fall into one of three categories: those in private practice; those employed by the "system" and in academic medical centers; those who are employed by the medical school as full-time faculty. The third and probably most important concept is that most physicians are very smart people. They would not have made it through medical school, residency, and achieved board certification if they were not intelligent. They usually have very good reasons for taking certain positions, even if you, as the leader, may not share that opinion. Finally, it is the job of the medical staff president to understand the priorities of the different groups and look for common ground. The common ground is, by and large, that each member of the medical staff wants to deliver high-quality medical care and wants the hospital to aid in their efforts.

In 1993, I relocated from Brooklyn to the Medical College of Pennsylvania (medical school and hospital), which was part of the Allegheny Health Education and Research Foundation. The Allegheny system was initially centered in Pittsburgh at Allegheny General Hospital. That institution had initial successes with its Cardiac Surgery and Trauma Services. Allegheny General Hospital thought that they needed their own medical school to help win their competition with the University of Pittsburgh. The Medical College of Pennsylvania started in the mid-nineteenth century as the Female Medical School and later the Women's Medical School. It was a medical school dedicated to the education of women physicians at a time when there were few opportunities for women. When the entry of women to medical schools was liberalized across the country, Women's Medical School became the Medical College of Pennsylvania in 1977 [1].

I was initially recruited to be the chief of Trauma and Surgical Critical Care. The Chief Medical Officer at the time, Dr. Harry Gottlieb, a well-respected endocrinologist, thought that I would make a good future leader of the medical staff and mentored me. A few years later, I found myself the president-elect of the Medical Staff and, as mentioned above, started my term early when the then-current president became ill. During my term as President, the system developed severe financial difficulties, secondary to poorly managed rapid expansion. It eventually filed for bankruptcy. During the bankruptcy experience, I learned, via trial and error, to hone my skills as a "cat herder."

When the bankruptcy was announced, the medical staff was in a panic. Most of the docs were full-time faculty, but there were some busy private practitioners. The major issues during the bankruptcy for the medical staff were quite serious: Would we still have a hospital, jobs, and incomes? None of us had any experience with the bankruptcy process and had no understanding of what it could mean for us. My first action, as Medical Staff President, was to put together a group of physician representatives from each of the major factions of the medical staff. I included in the meeting the top dozen or so high-volume practitioners and representatives from emergency medicine, pathology, and radiology departments. I did not include department chairs or service chiefs.

The first meeting was a disaster as I listened to everyone trying to speak at once. The anxiety in the air was palpable. The conversations were chaotic with each faction speaking without really listening. Eventually, we learned to slow down and to listen. We decided that our first step would be to employ an attorney to explain our options in the bankruptcy court. Our Medical Staff treasury had about $125,000.00 in the bank. A committee member approached one of the top firms in the city of Philadelphia. He met with us and, after listening politely, informed us that as physicians, we had no official standing in the bankruptcy court. We were neither creditors nor debtors. Whatever our concerns regarding our ability to take care of our patients or feed our families, we would have no way to influence the outcome of the court proceedings or sale of the health care delivery system in the city of Philadelphia.

We consulted another, lower-profile attorney who specialized in medical staff issues. He explained the bankruptcy process and figuratively held our hands until the eventual sale of the assets of the hospitals to Tenet, a for-profit company, and the medical school joined Drexel University. His initial advice to us was to maximize our ability, as a medical staff, to communicate and function with a singular voice. To this end, we set up a newsletter to communicate and educate the medical staff. This newsletter explained the bankruptcy process to the entire medical staff and defined our sphere of influence. Any prospective buyer would need the medical staff to make the venture successful. For the medical school to have any chance of a successful future, they would need their faculty mostly intact. Of the five hospitals in the Allegheny system in the Philadelphia area, the MCPH medical staff was the most well-organized and a force to be dealt with as we successfully spoke with one voice.

The following represents one example. Coming out of bankruptcy, the Chair of the pathology department wanted to take his department into a private practice that he would lead. He only wanted to bring with him selected members and leave almost half the department unemployed. The faculty in the department were rightfully quite upset and asked me for advice. I had them meet with my special committee. Our suggestion was that the department members should invite the dean of the medical school to a meeting and explain the situation, stating in direct, clear language that they no longer had any confidence in their chair. That strategy worked! The chair, shortly thereafter, was "fired" by the Dean. I would like to believe that the support of the entire medical staff for the pathology department played a role in the prompt resolution of the issue.

Medical staff leaders will unfortunately have to deal with physician disciplinary issues. The key in dealing with this issue is to always do that which is the safest for patient care while providing for due process for the individual medical staff members. All medical staff have detailed bylaws and rules and regulations that must be followed to the letter to ensure due process. Most medical staffs have a Code of Professional Conduct that has been approved by the Medical Executive Committee and signed off by medical staff members at the time of appointment and re-appointment. If they do not have one, they should.

I found over the years, both as a medical staff president and later as Chief Medical Officer (CMO), that dealing with behavior issues or compliance with policy issues are best handled by identifying them as early as possible. Adverse outcomes of investigations by medical staff organizations are required to be reported to the state department of health organizations and to the federal government's National Practitioner Data Bank (NPDB). The NPDB [2] is a database of the Department of Health and Human Services that holds reports of medical malpractice and negative findings such as healthcare criminal convictions, decisions made by certifying and licensing organizations. The database is available to authorized users such as hospitals and state boards.

Having private meetings with the practitioner as an intervention is the best method to avoid escalation to a formal reportable process (such as the NPDB). These meetings can be held as small group meetings: the practitioner with the medical staff president and another leader such as the CMO or service chief in attendance. It is important to have a witness present. These informal meetings need to be documented with notes placed in the practitioner's medical staff file. The documentation will prove to be crucial if a pattern of similar troubling issues develops. If the problem remains unresolved over time after multiple interventions, it will need to be brought before the Medical Executive Committee.

Any issue that affects patient safety or disrupts the smooth functioning of the hospital needs to be dealt with immediately, even if it requires emergency meetings of the Medical Executive Committee. Issues related to alcohol and drug use, grossly unsafe delivery of care, and lack of trainee supervision fit into this category. Unfortunately, I have had to deal with all these issues. I found following the medical staff bylaws closely, involving the medical staff's legal counsel when necessary, is essential.

The Medical Staff President must always remain impartial and treat everyone equally. If the involved physician is personally close to the medical staff president, such as a partner, friend, or relative or has a history with the individual practitioner, the medical staff president should recuse himself or herself from voting in or influencing the process.

Lessons Learned for Success as a Medical Staff Officer

1. Medical staff leadership, especially the medical staff president, must realize that they represent the entire medical staff. This may frequently be challenging. The medical staff is a pleomorphic group with multiple disciplines and factions. The president of the medical staff should keep in mind that the eyes of the medical staff are on him 24/7, and he/she needs to demonstrate excellence of character

continuously. It requires the ability to lead up, lead down, and particularly importantly lead sideways with your peers, and the other members of the medical staff. When dealing with conflicting priorities between factions, if the medical staff president has a reputation for fairness and always doing the best for patient care, he or she will tend to be forgiven by the disappointed faction. It is appropriate to build consensus and not rush major decisions that do not have an immediate direct effect on patient care. The medical staff president should not retreat from difficult, thorny issues. It is part of the job.

2. Listening to medical staff concerns and looking for the common ground that improves patient care is critical.
3. Leading in dealing with issues related to medical staff professionalism is frequently very challenging. The key is to treat everyone equally. This demonstration of integrity legitimizes a process inherent in difficult decisions. Early intervention before a process is initiated that warrants reporting to the National Practitioner Data Bank or state agencies is the best way to both safeguard patient care and the future of the practitioner. Strictly following the medical staff bylaws is essential.

References

1. Peitzman SJ. A new and untried course: Women's medical college and medical college of Pennsylvania. New Brunswick: Rutgers University Press; 2000.
2. National Practitioner Data Base (NPDB) (www.npdb.hrsa.gov).

Chapter 11
Branching Out into Hospital Leadership: Administration: Service Chief

Most service chiefs are usually remunerated for their administrative responsibilities by the hospital. Medical school faculty will frequently see that remuneration is filtered through the medical school and have it included in the total package of the individual's salary. Employed physicians are usually paid for that portion as part of the total salary support. Service Chiefs in private practice are usually paid directly just for that role. The job description for service chiefs usually includes leading the service efforts for performance improvement and regulatory compliance requirements.

Service leadership requires, like all medical leadership, emotional intelligence, character, and the realization that all eyes are on the leader all the time. I served as the Surgical Service Chief at Robert Wood Johnson University Hospital for 18 years. That hospital had a pleomorphic surgical service with a mixture of full-time faculty and private practitioners. I was a full-time faculty. At one point in time, the anesthesia service chief, after dealing with yet another behavioral issue on his service, was very frustrated. He thought that I appeared perpetually unscathed and asked me if I was "made of Teflon." He wanted to know why I was never given grief by hospital administration about my service's medical staff. I believe that the answer was straightforward. As I settled in and was no longer the "new guy," I had established a reputation for treating everyone the same. I dealt with issues as soon as they were identified and followed the lesson I learned as a Trauma Director: Always document closing the loop. Deal with issues in real time, document the conclusion, and feedback on the resolution.

Early on, I had to deal with an incident in the operating room of culturally inappropriate behavior allegedly committed by one of the hospital's division chiefs. This gentleman was also a division chief at the medical school and Vice-Chair of the Department of Surgery at the medical school. The first thing I did was to expeditiously start an investigation. I interviewed the nurses in the operating room who witnessed the exchange as well as the other direct participants. This was done in private. I did find that there were culturally insensitive remarks made by the division

S. Z. Trooskin, *An Introduction to Medical Leadership for Surgeons*, https://doi.org/10.1007/978-3-031-44264-3_11

chief. I took notes for my files. I counseled the service chief. A second investigation was carried out by the medical school after I informed them of the issue. I put together a Surgical Grand Rounds presentation on cultural sensitivity and appropriate behavior for the entire Surgical Service. I was demonstrating that I would not play favorites and would do the right thing, no matter who was involved.

Unfortunately, over the years, I dealt with other issues of rude and violent behaviors, surgeons who threw instruments or used inappropriate, insulting language, or exhibited misogynistic behavior. There were issues related to substance abuse, questionable trainee supervision, and technical and judgement competencies. The strategy that I learned via trial and error was to follow the algorithm of prompt response with early investigation. Copious documentation is essential, including liberal use of making notes to file. After the investigation is completed, it is important to take prompt appropriate action.

I also had to pay the price for doing my job well. One of my long-time friends, a member of my division, had repeated events related to inappropriate outbursts in the operating room and on the hospital floors. This was a person who was an excellent surgeon, someone who I personally trained and then hired to be my associate. We practiced together. Our families interacted socially for decades. Nonetheless, I investigated and met with him after every single one of the events. The behavioral issues seemed to be based on good intentions and concern for his patients, but his responses to stress escalated things and were counterproductive. I had notes for every meeting, which stayed in my files. I suggested on numerous occasions that he seek outside help, professional intervention, such as anger management or coaching. I thought that if he did not rectify his issues, his career would be in jeopardy. I told him of my concerns repeatedly. He did not take the advice, and the unacceptable behaviors were repeated over a very long time. When it reached the level of the Medical Executive Committee, I had to recuse myself from voting because of our personal relationship. He eventually lost his medical staff privileges. He attempted to bring a lawsuit and named me as one of the defendants. Although the lawsuit did not get very far, it did end our friendship.

Sometimes a service chief must deal with complicated quality initiatives that will require standardized behaviors from a multitude of providers. One such effort for me was the Surgical Care and Improvement Project (SCIP) [1]. There was an initiative to standardize the administration of prophylactic antibiotics to decrease postoperative wound infections. A national coalition of surgical leaders decided it was low-hanging fruit that, if adopted, would theoretically rapidly improve surgical outcomes. Specifically, it became a requirement to administer the appropriate antibiotics within an hour before making the skin incision. The thought process was that if there were high tissue levels of the right antibiotic, the incidence of wound infection would of course decrease. Being an initiative of the Centers for Medicare and Medicaid Services (CMS) compliance was mandatory.

This effort began within the first few years after I returned to Robert Wood University Hospital. My initial reaction was to be skeptical that this simplistic approach would in reality decrease the incidence of wound infections. I was convinced that preventing wound infections was much more complicated than just delivering timely antibiotics. There were multiple factors that could potentially affect the incidence of wound infections. These include patient factors, such as immune competency, diabetes, and nutritional status. The location of the operative site also affects the risk of infection. Colon operations have a high incidence of infection, while for thyroid operations the incidence is very low. There are bacteriologic factors as well. The virulence and quantity of the microbes are important.

I was given my assignment, which was to make sure that surgeons ordered the appropriate antibiotics on time. The memo went out to remind the surgeons to order the antibiotics on-call to the OR. Immediately, multiple functional problems came to light. Ordering the antibiotics on-call worked nicely for the first case of the day. For cases on the OR schedule listed as "to-follow," an on-call order was a recipe for failure. Since the to-follow cases had an unpredictable start time, the antibiotics were given frequently after the magic 1-hour window before incision time. This led to a high non-compliance rate. We decided to change the delivery time and to give the antibiotic when the patient was on the operating room table, just before making the skin incision. Doing it this way, the anesthesiologists would give the antibiotic and document administration by recording the time of delivery in the OR record. This proposal was met by pushback from our anesthesiology colleagues. We were asking them, yet again, to take on more work and responsibility. I could understand their concerns, but there was no other way to obtain improved compliance. We developed a tally of compliance/non-compliance and a provider feedback system. Compliance then improved somewhat.

At that time, the Chief of the Anesthesia Service and the Vice President for Perioperative Services were under ever-increasing pressure from the highest levels in the Administrative Suite to improve compliance. They were not able to move the needle further. There were several consistent anesthesiologists that remained outliers. I then took the rather dramatic step of sending a memo to the outlier anesthesiologists with my signature and sending a copy to the Dean of the medical school. Since all the anesthesiologists were full-time faculty, the compliance shortly thereafter approached 100%. And yes, the anesthesiologists did not appreciate my latest efforts of involving the Dean and let me know it quite vociferously. I survived those conversations and learned that one can make great progress by building consensus but sometimes a little negative reinforcement is necessary!

My experience with the SCIP issue was enlightening for me when attempting to deal with major issues that require large group behavioral changes. Individual leaders can attempt to move the process along, but a combined multidisciplinary effort will carry more weight. It will also spread the responsibility to more than one individual working solo. I believed that to adequately deal with this situation and to improve our ability to meet the future challenges of initiatives like SCIP, we needed to build an infrastructure for quality improvement that would combine the strengths of leadership of the Surgical Services, the Anesthesia Services, and the Perioperative Nursing Service. We created a Peri-operative Performance Improvement Committee and included representation from all the Services. We purposely selected very opinionated individuals and high-volume surgeons as opposed to division chiefs to serve on our committee. We were then positioned to deal more effectively and efficiently with issues such as retained foreign bodies, surgical site markings, instituting pre-procedural time-outs, and just about every quality initiative from that point forward.

Lessons Learned for Effective Leadership as a Service Chief

1. The most important behavior is to treat everyone equally. Investigate all issues as soon as possible.
2. You should document discussions for the file. Take actions that fit with the established policies and procedures.
3. Keep in mind that building consensus is preferable, but if the goal is imperative and attempts at consensus have failed, there are times when negative reinforcement is unavoidable. Teddy Roosevelt said: "Walk softly but carry a big stick."
4. As a Surgical Service leader, one must be able to articulate the mission of the institution and to lead up, sidewise, and down, always demonstrating character and emotional intelligence.

Reference

1. Surgical Care Improvement Project (SCIP) (www.ncbi.nim.nih.gov)

Chapter 12
Branching Out into Hospital Leadership: Administration: Chief Medical Officer

I served as Chief Medical Officer (CMO) at two hospitals, Medical College of Pennsylvania Hospital and Robert Wood Johnson University Hospital. During both tenures, I served in times of crisis. At the Medical College of Pennsylvania Hospital, the health care system underwent bankruptcy, and more recently at Robert Wood Johnson University Hospital during the global COVID-19 pandemic. The CMO is the hospital administration's physician representative to the staff. The medical staff recognizes this relationship. The CMO should strive to maintain the respect and credibility of the medical staff. The path to success is to always be honest in your dealings with the medical and nursing staff. There are times when the aspirations of the hospital administration will be contrary to the desires of the medical staff. The role of the CMO in this situation is to be the honest broker of information for both sides.

The CMO must deal openly with the hospital administration, even if it is not what they want to hear. Over the long run, it will be protective of everyone's best interests. Disagreements with the CEO and other administration leaders should be aired in private. The bottom line for the CMO is, above all else, to always do whatever is in the best interests of patient care. If the CMO does not follow this advice, he/she will lose credibility and will not last in the job. If the compromising of basic values is necessary to retain the position, the job is not worth having. On a certain level, I think that CEOs of hospitals may prefer their CMOs to blindly do their bidding. They would generally like to see their wishes become commands with expeditious carrying out of orders. Although the CEO may desire this, it may not always be in their best interest to achieve short-term success, when in the long-term failure will result. The CMO will have to be able to deliver bad news to his boss and to the medical staff. In my experience, this is unavoidable. The only way for the CMO to survive these inevitable conflicts is to be seen by all sides as an honest broker.

I have always believed that the CMO job should always be considered a temporary one. It is analogous to being a manager of a major league baseball team. Except for two notable long-tenured exceptions, Walter Alston and Tommy Lasorda, all

S. Z. Trooskin, *An Introduction to Medical Leadership for Surgeons*, https://doi.org/10.1007/978-3-031-44264-3_12

baseball managers get replaced without a decades long career. (Connie Mack, the long-term manager of the Philadelphia Athletics, does not count because he owned the team.) A relatively short career is a fact of life for most CMOs. Anyone taking this job needs to accept that this job may very well end sooner than later. The time frame may be unknown unless the CMO is at the end of their career. The CMO job can end because of the natural tension that may develop between a CMO and some CEOs that gets magnified over time. The CEO may want to remove the CMO because the CMO is unable to complete reasonable tasks. The projects that he/she has been assigned may not progress to completion or are not progressing at a fast enough rate. The CMO may be a bad fit with the rest of the administrative team or does not relate or interact with the medical staff leadership in a conducive way. The CMO may be terminated because of a change of hospital administration and the new CEO wants his "own people." My last CMO position ended because of this circumstance.

Acceptance of the knowledge that this is most likely a temporary position is crucial when making career decisions. There are several strategies to ensure that working as the CMO is not a dead-end career move. One strategy is not to give up "your day job." Remaining an active clinician while being the CMO has several salutary effects. Being active clinically allows for added credibility with the medical and nursing staff. It can preserve a safe landing zone after the term of CMO ends; it is an insurance policy for the future. You can always go back to being a full-time clinician. The other strategy is to become a CMO at the end of your career. Those individuals bring a wealth of experience to the job, and there is little risk if it does not work out as the next stop is a well-deserved retirement. I have used both of those strategies. I never felt like I was being held captive by having to preserve my job security when deciding the correct course of action. It was liberating to be able to work under those conditions.

I have worked with CEOs who demonstrated multiple styles of leadership, including the dogmatic, authoritative style, transformative style, and even toxic leader. I did have the pleasure of working with one CEO, Mr. John Gantner, who welcomed a contrary view and was not afraid to change his mind. He was the CEO who hired me as CMO at Robert Wood Johnson University Hospital, 6 months before the start of the pandemic in September of 2019. John had spent most of his career in the finance side of hospital administration. He had worked as the RWJUH CFO during its rapid growth phase during the 1990s through to the early 2000s. He left the hospital after the selection of a new CEO but returned in about 2018 as a consultant shortly after the merger of RWJ and Barnabas Systems. He was later appointed RWJUH CEO to deal with a financial deficit and falling public quality scores. John has a self-effacing yet gregarious personality. He frequently seemed to be ahead of the curve and thought "outside the box" when dealing with new situations. His Senior Leadership Meetings were a study in transformative leadership. These were held on Monday afternoons and frequently lasted over 2 hours. Ideas were discussed and vetted as a group. John would frequently bring up ideas he had and allow a free discussion with input from the group. He was not afraid to retreat from tentative plans when the group pointed out issues that he had not considered.

He dealt with this in a good-natured humorous way. The process of decision-making in the group was almost always via a vetting process before making a major decision. These decisions were frequently at odds with the system leadership, which led to conflicts with them. John always treated his team and me with respect, which was reciprocated. He also taught me how to do my job effectively.

Within 6 months of my starting this CMO position, we were faced with the COVID pandemic. In February 2020, we began to prepare our responses to the pandemic. We were faced, as was every other hospital in the world, with little concrete information. The guidelines from the CDC were continually changing, at times it seemed by the hour. One of my first assignments was to lead the efforts to create the medical manpower component of our surge plan to deal with the projected increasing influx of COVID patients. With the cooperative efforts of the Chairs of the departments of Medicine, Surgery, and Anesthesiology, this was accomplished rather easily.

Like many hospitals in New York and New Jersey, in March of 2020 we had to decide the timing of redistributing Operating Room Staff to care for more COVID patients. That effort was coordinated with the process of triaging surgical patients needing the operating room. We had to prioritize emergency operations for the most serious conditions. Some decisions were easy: Acutely injured patients and those with immediate life or limb-threatening conditions obviously needed immediate access to the operating room. Purely elective operations such as those for joint replacement or morbid obesity could be safely delayed for the short term. The decision to delay operations for cancer patients or perform cardiac catheterization was more difficult. I found those decisions much more challenging in terms of the distribution of resources to manage the deluge of patients presenting with respiratory compromise from COVID-19 infections. Mr. Gantner stayed involved with these major decisions. At the beginning of this process, my medical leadership colleagues and I tended to be overly strict in limiting access to the operating room. John helped us modulate this so we could continue to take care of more cancer patients needing operations and other procedures that, if we could avoid it, should not be delayed. He attended the triage meetings that I ran to monitor our efforts and track delayed patients. He helped the Chairs of Anesthesia and Surgery and me as we developed the protocols that we eventually applied to the first and then to the next two COVID surges. I found it remarkable that he helped me with this politically charged process without resorting to criticism as I struggled to do my best with these difficult decisions. Throughout the pandemic, I learned from him how to reset processes as needed under dire circumstances.

There was a shortage of PPE (personal protective equipment) from the early days of the pandemic and throughout the first wave. We, like other institutions, developed ways to conserve our PPE and stay within the ever-changing CDC guidelines. As expected, our staff remained appropriately very anxious about having enough of the right PPE. Protection of our staff was a top priority. Thinking again "out of the box," John had our CFO order reusable heavy-duty industrial masks that we could fit with the correct medical grade air filters. We had them sequestered if we needed them in the future. Although we did not need these ugly rubber masks, knowing that we had them ready to use and had the ability, on hand, to protect our staff was comforting for the senior leadership.

John also started planning for our bounce back to normal hospital functioning at the height of the first surge. He knew that we had to be ready to handle the increase in procedural volume and to deal with the lag in some services to return to pre-pandemic levels. When the time came to resume elective work, we were ready! John Gantner was out in front of all our preparations for the COVID pandemic including our bounce back plan to normal functioning. We were far ahead of the rest of our system with our plans. We had the earliest return to full service in our hospital system.

Expectation Management for CMOs

It is critical for the CMO to manage the expectations of the administrative team where they intersect with the practice of medicine and patient care. When given an assignment by the CEO, the CMO should study the problem and then provide feedback on his or her opinions regarding the feasibility of the task. At frequent intervals, the CMO should update the administrative team on the progress of the project and get input from them. Barriers and time frames need to be presented.

One of the CMO's responsibilities should be to serve as the medical educator to the administrative team. The CEO may at times be bombarded by experts such as division chiefs or department chairs lobbying for their programs. It frequently will be up to the CMO to understand and explain the long- and short-term advantages and disadvantages of the various programs and where they align with the institution's or system's priority list. Surprises will inevitably come up while managing complex institutions, like a medical center. The CMO should not be adding more surprises. Keeping everyone on the administrative team and specifically the CEO involved with updates is critical in managing expectations.

Project Management for CMOs

I found that keeping track of all my projects, the progress and the next steps, was quite challenging. At one point, I had a project list that numbered well over 25. To handle these, I used an application on my computer and the small tablet that I carried with me to all my meetings. I worked closely with my administrative assistant, who also had access to the program. There are a number of these apps that are commercially available. I preferred one that allowed me to upload/scan in related paperwork. I included all my notes for meetings in the different "chapters" that I created. Each major project had an assigned chapter. Once a week, I updated my progress and planned the next steps on the highest priority items. I could also move projects up or down my priority list. My practice of weekly project review allowed me to determine which ones were stalled and needed my attention. If I had assigned the responsibility for a given task and I had not received feedback with a progress report, I could therefore be reminded to make the inquiry and investigate. It also protected me from just focusing on the latest crisis or crises. I did not want to be blindsided by a question of status on any of my projects.

It is critical to understand the institutional priorities that will become your priorities. What will become your marching orders, and in what order will you pursue them? I found that this was simple to do by attending the appropriate meetings and listening carefully. These meetings include the Hospital Board of Director meetings, Medical Executive Committee meetings, and Senior Leadership Meetings. I used my one-on-one meetings with the CEO to make sure that my priority list coincided with the CEO's. I also used the CEO meetings to update my progress on the various projects and to seek consultation on how better to proceed.

The Hospital Board of Directors may vary in how they carry out their fiduciary responsibilities. Some Boards may be intimately involved in the operations of the institution, while others that I have experienced just go through the motions. Either way, the Hospital Board of Directors meetings were very important for me. As the CMO, I did not have a vote but was considered staff. The President of the Medical Staff is usually a voting member of this Board. Most Hospital Boards are composed of community leaders, successful businesspeople, or retired successful businesspeople. As I remember it, the Allegheny Health and Research Foundation Board seemed to me to be populated, in the 1990s, with board members, who were a rubber stamp for whatever the system CEO, Shariff Abdelhak, wanted.

I remember one meeting that occurred shortly before the bankruptcy was declared. An outside financial audit report, which was over 100 pages, was handed out and collected approximately 10 mins later. I could only read a few pages before it was collected. There was a topic on the meeting agenda for discussion that was quite shocking. It was a proposal, suggested and then approved, to sell the hospital parking deck and convert that funding to cover operational losses! I was quite naive at the time and did not understand that this weak Board had abrogated their fiduciary responsibilities. I should not have been surprised that filing for bankruptcy followed shortly after that meeting.

At Robert Wood Johnson University Hospital, the Board of Directors had members who were involved in the nitty-gritty of the hospital's business. They had members who read every word of the minutes of the Executive Medical Board meetings, including the addendums. Small details were brought up for discussion as they saw all this information well in advance of the meeting. They delved into the details of the official reports on quality and asked probing questions. They wanted to know the plans for remediation. When no improvement was noted, they did not hesitate to vocalize their concerns. I learned the Board's priorities needed to also be my priorities, whether it was overtly stated or not. I believed that I was at risk for being responsible for the Board's highest priorities.

One of the major responsibilities of the CMO is the quality program. When there is another physician assigned by the CEO as being responsible for the Quality Program, the CMO will nonetheless be the one assumed to have been responsible. I also observed incidences in the national media that covered the very public and scandalously poor outcomes. These frequently resulted in the dismissal of the CMO, because in terms of quality, the CMO is the ultimate responsible physician. One of my former surgical residents was the CMO of a major university medical center. He was trained, in addition to general surgery, in complex surgical oncology. The scandal in that medical center involved poor outcomes in cardiac surgery program and issues in the hospital's Transfusion Services. These outcome results reached both the local and national media, where I first noted them. I was not privy to the specific details and responsibilities of the CMO at that medical center, but I do understand the usual CMO workflow. The CMO would ordinarily work with the subspecialty experts to formulate plans for improvement. That academic medical center had a historical reputation for excellence in cardiac surgery, and I suspect the resources were present for eventual improvement. Once the problems hit the national press, the CMO along with the CEO and CNO lost their jobs. All CMOs should assume that they can be held responsible for quality failures.

I have seen similar events play out with the same result; that is, the CMO "takes the hit" among others, for poor outcomes or other scandalous issues, if they reach the news cycle. It is one of the reasons that I concluded that the CMO position is very far from a long-term appointment and those taking that position need to realize this phenomenon.

Lessons Learned to be Effective as a Chief Medical Officer

1. The CMO position is a time-limited responsibility. Anyone choosing to do this should understand this and have a plan for the next step in their career. As a rule, clinicians should stay clinically active. It is their insurance policy to put food on their table.
2. The CMO position requires the execution of daily emotional intelligence. It requires expertise in leading up, sideways, and down. The CMO must work closely with other members of the administrative team especially the CEO (leading up). Controlling expectations by excellent and frequent communication is essential. The CMO, with a lot of help from the CNO, is responsible for educating the lay part of the administrative team. The CMO, in the role as staff to Board of the Directors, needs to understand their priorities and be prepared to address them.
3. The CMO is the hospital administration liaison to the medical staff. This leading sideways must be done with complete transparency for the CMO to retain credibility and help move the agenda forward. Listening and understanding the issues of the diverse medical staff is critical. One does not always have to agree, as there is always a place for honest disagreement. One does have to listen and consider. The CMO must always take the high ground as the advocate for patient care.

4. Leading down, the CMO must make real progress on assigned projects and work closely with service chiefs to move the needle. Efficient project management is a major key to success. Choosing the right clinical leader to help lead projects is very important. This is Collins's getting the right people in the right seats on the bus. The more multidisciplinary the team, the greater the likelihood of success. Keeping a list of all the activities and projects is very helpful as is reviewing them for progress weekly.

Chapter 13
When It is Time to Go

There are several reasons to move on to a new position. Career advancement is one of the best reasons for leaving a current role. The current position may have been planned as just a step up the ladder, and a better opportunity now presents itself. Feeling chronically frustrated at the lack of progress or lack of support may be another reason. Sometimes a leadership position that looked so good from afar does not seem the right fit after arrival and having actual experience. Leaders can also be asked to leave. It could also be that it is time to leave for a combination of reasons. I have experienced most of these reasons for leaving.

I left Robert Wood Johnson University Hospital in 1989 after being recruited to be the Chief of Trauma at the Kings County Hospital Center. It was not a lateral move but a career advancement to have the opportunity to lead a major trauma center and an opportunity to join a larger department with a higher national profile. Admittedly, I had spent 9 years trying to develop a level 1 Trauma Center and was somewhat tired of the daily institutional frustrations and ready to deal with new challenges. The move to Philadelphia was also a step up, as was my return as Chief of Surgical Services to Robert Wood Johnson in 2002. Both of those were career advances, but there were other factors involved. My department in Brooklyn imploded after 3 years, and in Philadelphia I wanted to escape the aftermath of the bankruptcy. I believe that my last position as a CMO ended as the new CEO wanted to recruit his own person "to go in a different direction."

Whatever the reasons, there are certain recommendations that can be made about leaving. First, keep in mind that the worlds of those in surgical or in medical administration are small, tight-knit communities where no secrets are kept for long. There are only a few degrees of separation between Chairs of Surgery. They all know each other or know someone who knows someone. If you interview for a position at an outside institution, it will be common knowledge at the home base in very short order. The best strategy to take is to inform your immediate superior, Chief, Chair, Dean, or CEO that you were asked to interview for a position. Do this well before the interview. If you are relatively happy with your current position, do not hesitate to let your boss know. Keep them involved in the process of your recruitment. If they value you and your efforts, they will not want to see you leave and will have time to prepare a nice, competitive counteroffer. Giving them the courtesy of your honesty will allow them to prepare an offer to sweeten your prospects of staying. When I have suggested this to some faculty, they have expressed the fear that investigating a new position will be looked at as an act of disloyalty. My response is that sneaking around and having it heard secondhand is the real action demonstrating disloyalty and disrespect.

When you are going through the recruitment process, never make an ultimatum to your present boss unless you are ready to leave and therefore have nothing to lose. It is important to be in control of the process as much as possible. I have been in a situation where my response to one of my people, who gave me an ultimatum or had outrageous demands, was to congratulate them and politely wish them well with their new opportunity.

It is a good idea to continue to carry yourself with dignity during the process of deciding whether to leave or after having made the decision to leave. Your character is always on display, and if you leave in anger, making disparaging public outbursts, and badmouthing the institution while you leave, that reputation will follow you to your next position. When I accepted the position as Chief of Trauma at Kings County, I continued to work hard until the day I left Robert Wood Johnson University Hospital. I took excellent care of my patients and transitioned their care to my colleagues. When asked why I was leaving, I focused on describing the opportunity that lay ahead for me, and I did not include whatever was responsible for my pent-up frustrations. I continued to represent Robert Wood Johnson University Hospital publicly, at state-wide meetings, to open the trauma center designation process. Leaving on good terms, I believe allowed me the luxury of returning 13 years later as Chief of the Surgical Services.

Lessons Learned for Successful Leaving

1. Continue to act as the responsible transformative leader demonstrating character. Use your emotional intelligence, transfer your responsibilities the best you can, and hold your head up high and behave with dignity.

Chapter 14
Final Thoughts

Medicine today needs leaders who understand clinical care and are also dedicated to improving patient access and outcomes. The characteristics that today lead to excellence in clinical practice are like those needed for excellence in administrative leadership. Emotional intelligence with a constant demonstration of character excellence is the key to success in clinical practice and medical leadership. Learning to maximize interpersonal skills and relationships is essential for success. Understanding what went wrong and what will work better next time is an essential trait. Surgeons start preparing for leadership early in their training via active participation in M&M Conferences. Surgeons, by the nature of what they do and the daily responsibilities they carry out, taking care of patients, building practices, and leading teams in the Operating Rooms, have routinely learned leadership via trial and error. Although leadership training will always involve trial and error with self-correction, more directed leadership training and mentorship may very well prevent some of those errors.

Courses in medical leadership are tremendous assets for leadership training. I found the leadership course I took late in my career to be very helpful. I realized that most of what I had learned was by trial and error. This is not an efficient method for training future medical leaders. In this book, I attempted to focus on leadership training involving interpersonal interactions, at the various career levels of residency, junior attending, clinical practice, and program building. The roles of division, department, or hospital administration leadership can be very challenging, and there are few or no specific courses to help develop those leaders. To try to fill some of those gaps, I attempted to focus on the different career stages, using my own trial and error experiences to underscore the specific lessons regarding emotional intelligence that I found to be important. I tried to link those personal lessons to the leadership lessons offered in the classic medical leadership courses. I hope you found this somewhat helpful.

© The Author(s), under exclusive license to Springer Nature Switzerland AG 2023
S. Z. Trooskin, *An Introduction to Medical Leadership for Surgeons*, https://doi.org/10.1007/978-3-031-44264-3_14

Index